THE
ESSENTIAL
OILS
BOOK

CREATING PERSONAL BLENDS
FOR MIND & BODY

COLLEEN K. DODT

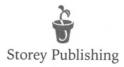

Storey Publishing

The mission of Storey Publishing is to serve our customers by publishing practical information that encourages personal independence in harmony with the environment.

Edited by Deborah L. Balmuth
Cover and text design and production by Carol J. Jessop, Black Trout Design
Cover and text illustrations © John Nelson/Represented by Irmeli Holmberg
How-to line drawings by Brigita Fuhrmann
Indexed by Northwind Editorial Services

The information in this book is true and complete to the best of our knowledge. All recommendations are made without guarantee on the part of the author or Storey Publishing. The author and publisher disclaim any liability in connection with the use of this information. For additional information please contact Storey Publishing, 210 MASS MoCA Way, North Adams, MA 01247.

Storey books are available for special premium and promotional uses and for customized editions. For further information, please call 1-800-793-9396.

Printed in the United States by Versa Press
30 29 28 27 26 25 24 23 22 21 20

Library of Congress Cataloging-in-Publication Data

Dodt, Colleen K., 1955–
      The essential oils book : creating personal blends for mind & body /
      Colleen K. Dodt.
             p.   cm.
      Includes bibliographical references and index.
      ISBN 978-0-88266-913-7 (pbk. : alk. paper)
      1. Aromatherapy — Popular works.   I. Title.
RM666.A68D63   1996
615'.321— dc20   95-39021
                                              CIP

TABLE OF CONTENTS

He is happiest who hath the power to gather wisdom from a flower.
— Mary Howitt, circa 1825

For the sweetest flower I know,
my dear daughter Christina Kaye Dodt

ACKNOWLEDGMENTS

A heartfelt thanks to friends, family, work-study students, and strangers who have believed in my herbal endeavors and encouraged me to believe in myself.

Thank you to Storey Communications, Inc. for allowing me to share some of my journey.

Thanks to Mr. Lawrence E. Dove, II for the kind generosity and encouragement that helped me to make this book a reality, and to, Mr. Gary Wanttaja of Nature's Products and Ms. Sandra Hazel of Word Works Literary Services for their computer expertise and calm, professional direction on those difficult days when I truly believed computers and printers should be given flying lessons.

To my parents, Marie E. Marker and the late Frederick P. Marker, my thanks for LIFE and the drive to live it to its fullest.

To Ollie and George, the parents God gave me, my sincere love, respect, and thanks for connecting me with the earth through their generous, holistic outlook on life.

And to the the plants that produce pure essential oils themselves, my life's essentials, I offer humble gratitude and deepest respect.

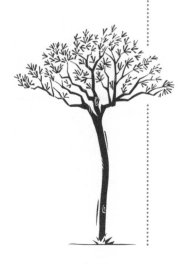

PREFACE

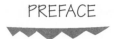

Herbs and pure essential oils have been an intimate part of my life for 15 years. Being involved with aromatic plants on a daily basis has instilled in me an insatiable quest for knowledge about the aromatic substances that give flowers and herbs their marvelous scents.

I have been intrigued with this "life force" or essential spirit of plants from the very first time I crushed sprigs of peppermint, lavender, and other fragrant herbs between my fingers and experienced the delightful fragrance that fills the air. When I started my herbal education, very little literature was available on the subject. I contacted essential oil suppliers, experimented, traveled to England, and researched every source available. The information I gathered has been woven into an ongoing education that continues to excite and delight me daily.

Recently, the use of pure essential oils has gained popularity as a result of renewed interest in the art of aromatherapy. Essential oils are being promoted in body-care products, medicinal mixtures, beauty products, and to enhance one's personal environment. Yet, there are still many opinions as to what aromatherapy entails. There is very little standardized education, or qualifications recognized in the United States. There are schools and correspondence courses available, but most are either weekend courses or short-term residential programs, rather than degree programs. The term aromatherapy seems to be taken more seriously in Europe, in general, and in England especially where approximately 25 schools and more than one professional association are now active in the pursuit of essential oil education and aromatherapy definition.

I define aromatherapy as the use of pure essential oils to enhance the quality of body, mind, and spirit. Many Americans still confuse the use of pure essential oils with any type of scented oil. Reading this book, you will soon realize that scented oils do not have the same effect as pure essential oils. There is a great group of people internationally who have devoted lifetimes and careers to the research of aromatic substances. Through these dedicated folks, everyone will soon have access to knowledge in the use of pure essential oils and aromatherapy.

I believe we have just started to explore all the possibilities for incorporating the use of essential oils into our lives, even though their history is ancient. For early humans, the sense of smell was a survival tool that served them well. Scent is a language that almost every living thing speaks and understands. People in ancient Egyptian and Roman societies refined the art of using aromatic plants, woods, fruits, herbs, flowers, spices, and resins to enhance their moods, prayers, and homes. More recently, the glove makers of old Europe often impregnated their wares with scented oils to ward off insects and the stench of foul streets through which the wearers traveled. The European tradition of carrying nosegays or tussie mussies was another attempt at aromatic protection. When one rubbed the leaves of aromatic plants, the pure essential oils contained in them were emitted into the air to help purify and protect the carrier. Canes or walking sticks were designed with tops that stored packed spices to inhale. These traditions provide a foundation for contemporary exploration of aromatherapy. As I wrote in an article entitled "Aroma What?" that appeared in *The International Journal Of Aromatherapy* in February 1988 (volume 1, number1), "We have much to learn from our European counterparts. But we learn fast and we are well on our way to another American Revolution — the Aromatic Revolution." Pure essential oils have a place in every home and every lifestyle. They are nature's alternative to the many synthetic chemicals that have invaded our lives and homes in the names of health, cleanliness, and environmental enhancement.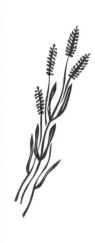

Unlike many other aromatherapy books available today that focus on the medicinal and spiritual use of essential oils, this book concentrates on the everyday uses of pure essential oils — simple easy ways to incorporate these precious substances into your life. I also provide you with straightforward information on the precautions that must be observed when incorporating these aromatic allies into your world. Within the covers of this book, I hope I offer enough information and enthusiasm to entice you to embark on your own further education and experimentation with herbs and pure essential oils. If you choose to go on and acquaint yourself with chemical constituents or massage techniques often associated with the term aromatherapy there are in-depth, quality publications to aid you in your quest.

It is my distinct pleasure to share the precious knowledge I have gained — the same knowledge that was used for centuries before the advent of synthetic aromatic chemicals. In this book, you will find recipes for experiences that can turn your world around, from sensual baths to naturally fresh-smelling carpets. Based on my experience with countless clients, customers, friends, and neighbors, I feel confident saying that there are pure essential oils that will enhance your life. One must only remember to take the time to stop and smell the roses, lemon, lavender, rosemary . . . .

Essentially yours,
Colleen K. Dodt
Rochester Hills, Michigan
February 1995

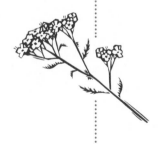

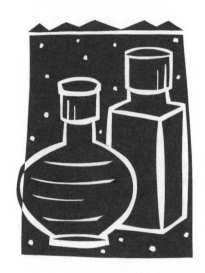

Awakening

the

Scent Sense

CHAPTER 1

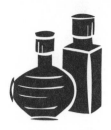

We often take our olfactory world for granted and, unless directly stimulated, ignore our sense of smell. Stop for a moment and reflect upon your personal sense of smell. Is it strong or weak? Which scents attract or repel you? Do you like floral, herbal, fruity, earthy, or spicy scents? What is your favorite scent? Your least favorite? Why do you like or dislike certain scents?

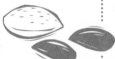

SMELL AND PERCEPTION

In his *Aromatherapy Workbook,* Marcel Lavabre notes that the French word *sentir* means "to smell, to feel." We "feel" scents, rather than logically think about them. There is very little language to describe scent. We understand it more through associations and images than by analytical processes or data. In the limbic portion of the brain, emotions and odors are directly linked and have been found to produce some of the same electrical impulses. The limbic system is also called the rhinencephalon, or "smell part" of the brain.

Smell plays a significant role in how we perceive places and situations. Good smells help us to feel good, bad ones depress us. Think about walking into a beautiful room, immaculate in every way. How would you feel about that room if it smelled terrible? Regardless of what you saw, the bad scent would make you uncomfortable. Likewise, imagine arriving at the door of the worst place you ever saw but, upon entering, discovering it smelled of roses. Your sense of smell would likely diminish your discomfort with the place, and make you a little more willing to explore it. Unless, of course, you have experienced a direct negative experience with the scent of roses in the past. Then your anxiety level may actually increase due to this previous scent-conditioning experience. People often associate the smell of a place such as a hospital, nursing home, or funeral home with what they experienced there. Although these places may do their best to create a clean or comfortable environment, people often have negative emotions tied to the time they spent there and to the scent they remember.

For many of us, the sense of smell is greatly diminished by sinus problems, pollution, and the synthetic aromatic chemicals we are bombarded with daily. These can reek havoc on our delicate sense of smell. I notice my sense of smell is always heightened after being closed in the steamy bathroom with aromatic essential oils. The additional heat and moisture in the air make the odor molecules more accessible to my nose. As I walk through the kitchen en route from the bathroom to the boudoir, scents in the house that usually go unnoticed suddenly come alive.

RETRAINING YOUR SENSE OF SMELL

I have often seen clients taken aback by the scent of pure undiluted essential oils. The oils are so strong that people don't know quite how to react. Our sense of smell often requires some retraining to appreciate natural scents. These oils, which require large amounts of plant material to produce, are very concentrated!

The next time you peel an orange, squeeze a lemon, apply your favorite perfume, or stop to savor the scent of a rose, think about what you are experiencing. Write down your reaction. Be aware of your olfactory world. We are truly led by the nose! Pure essential oils make this journey a wonderful adventure.

The fruit bowl is redolent with ripening bananas, pears, and oranges; the coffee grinder smells of good Kona coffee; the small bottle of my personal perfume on the bedroom dresser is sweet and familiar as I search for my clothes; and when I open the towel cupboard in the bathroom, the scent of line-dried towels fills my nostrils. Is there a scent to line-dried clothes? I say yes, but I couldn't say what it is comprised of — unless sun and wind have a scent of their own.

SCENT AS PROTECTION

On a misty spring day in late March when I went out to my mailbox, I noted the scent of celery that had been left in the garden over the winter. Heat, light, air, and moisture all activate the release of scent. Smell helps orient us to place, season, and even imminent danger.

For our ancestors the ability to find a mate, a home, or even the search for food depended greatly upon olfactory acuity. Even today we detect danger with our nose. If there is a gas leak at home, the scent added to natural gas will warn us very quickly. If some leftovers in the refrigerator have been there too long, our nose will tell us not to eat them. Poisonous plants often have a bad acrid smell that warns not to ingest them, while the sweet-scented herbs that can enhance our everyday existence invite us to consume them through the release of their oils. From the day we are born, our sense of smell is an intimate link to our survival.

People who suffer anosmia, meaning they have lost their sense of smell, are often prone to depression due to the lack of scent in their world. I received a letter from a man who had worked very diligently to improve his sense of smell. He said he could smell very clearly the ink with which he was writing the letter. He asserted that if more people had an alive sense of smell instead of an often deadened one, we would not be able to tolerate the stench of the society we live in today. I couldn't help but wonder how he would have adjusted to past times of open sewage in the streets and no garbage disposal!

For a strange twist on the sense of smell, read the novel *Perfume: The Story of a Murderer,* by Patrick Suskind. In this novel set in the French countryside, life and death hinges upon a keen, obsessive olfactory sense. Another interesting account of the sense of smell is *A Natural History of The Senses,* by Diane Ackerman. Ms. Ackerman explains how the sense of smell has guided us down the dimly lit corridors of evolution. The agony of anosmia is portrayed and examined.

USING SCENT TO PRODUCE PARTICULAR RESPONSES

The subliminal use of scent to produce particular behavioral responses is widespread in our society. Scratch-and-sniff entered our children's lives long ago, and magazines aren't complete today without a scented advertisement or two. Many products contain subliminal scenting of which consumers are often totally unaware. Think about this: Do you buy a product because it cleans well or because it smells like a refreshing lemon or a pine forest? A large car manufacturer approached me once to ask if I could create "new-car" smell. I told them they needed a chemist, not an essential oil consultant. Well, they promptly found one, and they now spray "new-car" smell in their used cars to enhance sales.

Neurochemical Experiences Produced by Essential Oils

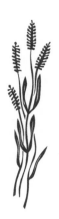

People say lavender smells clean. How can something smell clean? I know I can smell the scent of spring. I have also experienced scent in dreams. It is learned-odor responses — odors that have memories attached to them — that lead us on these olfactory emotional odysseys. Learned-odor responses arouse reactions to certain synthetic or natural scents, like the scent of an ex-lover's perfume or the smell of freshly mown grass.

However, our experience of a pure essential oil is different than a learned-odor response. When an essential oil is inhaled, various neurochemicals are released in the brain and the inhaler experiences a physiological change in body, mind, and spirit. When lavender is inhaled, for instance, serotonin is released from the raphe nucleus of the brain, producing a calming influence in the body. This effect is altered, however, if the inhaler has had a direct negative experience with lavender.

A learned-odor response can alter or interfere with the biochemical effects of essential oils. An intense emotional response to a certain odor may interfere with the chemical release from the brain. Emotions have their own chemical make-up and can be powerful enough to inhibit or enhance a neurochemical release or absorption. For this reason, over-the-counter aromatherapy formulas aren't effective for everyone, since people's life experiences are so varied. For example, if a child had a caretaker in their life who wore a certain scent such as lavender, a known relaxant, and that caretaker had a direct negative association for this particular child, it could perhaps be difficult for this person to relax when exposed to lavender because of a learned-odor response. In the same vein, an odor many find offensive, such as barnyard, may have a positive influence for one raised happily on a farm. Sweet orange essential oil has a generally uplifting association for some people.

Others find its effects sedative. However if one has had a direct negative experience associated with this scent — such as being forced to work long and hard to harvest this fruit — you may no longer find this scent uplifting or sedative at all. This association to sweet orange would be a learned-odor response. I am not acquainted with any direct research in overcoming or changing learned-odor responses with pure essential oils.

Chemical reproductions of pure essential oils don't hold this olfactory magic and are not effective in aromatherapy. They rely solely on learned-odor response, not neurochemical release. Chemical reproductions do not have the same biochemical effects as naturally occurring pure essential oils.

The effects of essential oils are both scientific and experiential. As you become more familiar with pure essential oils and the scents that surround you in your personal worlds, the experiential influences will be greatly enhanced. I have often been comforted by a familiar scent when I was miles away from home because I associated it with the comfort of home. The neurochemical releases influence our emotional response to various essential oils and the context in which they are employed.

I have a poster produced by Tisserand Aromatherapy, Ltd., in England, entitled *Psycho-Aromatherapy,* that details the various pure essential oils and how they affect the brain. The

---

THE HEALING EFFECTS OF ESSENTIAL OILS

When someone walks into my house they say, "Gee what smells so good?" It is amazing how I can see people visibly change when they come into contact with pure essential oils. Throughout history, people have believed in the healing effects of herbs. During times of plague, it was believed that the perfumers and glovers didn't fall ill because they were constantly exposed to the essential oils in their daily work. It was very fashionable to have one's gloves perfumed with pure essential oils. People also carried little nosegays or tussie mussies fashioned from freshly cut herbs and flowers. These little bouquets were held up to the nose while out in the streets in a time of, shall we say, less than adequate sanitation. The herbs and flowers, of course, contained pure essential oils. Why do you think bringing herbs and flowers to someone in the hospital started? Rosemary, thyme, and lavender herbs were burnt on hospital wards of long ago to help purify the air.

poster quotes Edward Sagarin, who in 1945 said, "Odour is the story of language, of man's efforts to find words to express emotion and sensation. It is allied with all the senses; indissolubly with taste, with colour, sound and memory, and deeply affected by the psychological phenomenon, the power of suggestion." In small print at the bottom, it says, "The above is scientifically proven." This, to me, captures the logical, yet mysterious, way in which our sense of smell, and our experience of essential oils, influences our world.

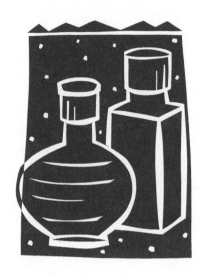

An Introduction
to Buying and
Using Pure
Essential Oils

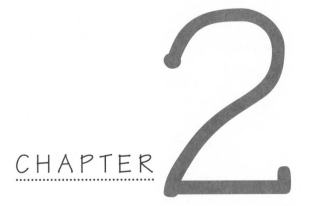

CHAPTER 2

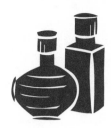

The term "essential oil" is thrown about every day, with a wide range of meanings. There are no standardized regulations for use of the words "essential oil" or "essence," so they are often used to describe any number of products which have little or nothing to do with the real thing or meaning.

When I refer to essential oils in this book I mean the pure plant distillates and extracts that are excellent allies in yesterday's, today's, and tomorrow's world of home health care. They are naturally derived, and should be respected as powerful substances to be used with caution and education. Pure essential oils are extracted directly from different parts of plants, depending on the oil concerned. Some are extracted from flowers, others from leaves, stems, the rind of fruit, berries, resin, or roots.

There are a variety of extraction methods, including distillation, expression, solvent extraction, effleurage, the phytonic process, and the super critical carbon dioxide extraction. The extraction process used depends on the plant. For example, orange, lemon, grapefruit, and bergamot are usually expressed because the oils are present in the peels and released when the peel is ruptured. Others, including lavender, clary sage, chamomile, and rose geranium, are distilled. Some flowers, like rose, are distilled and solvent

WHAT IS AN ESSENTIAL OIL?

Pure essential oils are some of life's greatest pleasures. Their name itself is indicative of their status in everyday life. Webster's dictionary, which is my favorite book, defines "essential" as: 1. Of or constituting the intrinsic, fundamental nature of something; basic; inherent. 2. Absolute; complete; perfect; pure. 3. Necessary to make a thing what it is; indispensable; requisite. 4. Containing or having the properties of a concentrated extract of a plant, drug or food. Essential oils are nature by the drop, to enjoy and enhance life. They contain the life force of a valuable botanical in a form that is basic and easy to access. Anything essential is absolutely necessary, a fundamental requisite to healthier living.

extracted, resulting in either a rose absolute or rose otto. The variety of rose used also makes a difference. Extraction of pure essential oils usually requires laboratory equipment and a large amount of materials for a small yield of oil. I have seen directions for homemade stills, yet found them too much bother for such a small yield. Distilling in a small ready-made still from Europe has helped me appreciate why many oils are expensive and can be difficult to locate. I, for one, will leave the extraction to those who know their business and be glad that I don't have to try to acquire my own oils by extracting them. My rosewater experience each summer is enough extraction for me, and for most home gardeners. If you are interested in trying extraction at home, you can find detailed information in some of the books listed in the appendix on page 145.

However it is extracted, the resulting oil is a highly concentrated, volatile substance that is made up of many different elements,

A WORD ON THE COST OF PURE ESSENTIAL OILS

I am truly grateful that there are people in the world dedicated to producing the plant material to extract pure essential oils. When I really think about how much time goes into producing the contents of one little brown bottle, I am better able to explain why they can be so costly. I, for one, am willing to pay the price of pure essential oils of the best quality.

As demand for aromatherapy-quality pure essential oils is made known, hopefully more people will realize the need to grow the material to produce them, which might make the oils more available and affordable. Sandalwood and rosewood trees are both being depleted and are in great need of being replanted. If we are to use these natural resources, we have a responsibility to replace them.

including alcohols, esters, hydrocarbons, aldehydes, ketones, phenols, terpene alcohols, and acids. Chemists have tried to recreate essential oils in the laboratory, but, to date, they have not been 100 percent successful.

BUYING PURE ESSENTIAL OILS

As a buyer, you must beware of imitations! Better yet, be educated! Synthetic aromatic chemicals have become the norm for so long that many folks are used to them, and are unaware of the choices they have from nature's bounty. Recently, I was in a very nice little shop full of scented goodies. I approached the essential oils section and found pretty little bottles with signs and labels indicating they were filled with essential oils and aromatherapy products. The slick-looking display covered with pictures of herbs and flowers led me to believe that these were indeed the true thing, but upon closer inspection I found that all the bottles were the same price. This is a clear tip-off that you're not dealing with pure essential oils since the prices of these precious oils vary greatly, depending on their accessibility and ease of extraction. I would love to find true jasmine absolute oil at the same price as lavender oil, but I don't think that will ever happen in my lifetime! Upon smelling the sampler in this shop, my suspicions that these were synthetic aromatic chemicals, not pure essential oils, were confirmed. The shopkeeper was shocked and dismayed at my discovery. She truly thought she was offering a quality aromatherapy product, and was not properly informed by her supplier.

I have happened across this same scene time and time again around the world. The adulteration, dilution, and imitation of pure essential oils has become big business — at the consumer's expense, both financially and ethically. However, with a little education and exposure to pure essential oils, you, too, will be able to sniff out the imposters.

LOOK FOR HIGH-QUALITY OILS

The quality of even pure essential oils can vary greatly depending on the country where the plant was grown, climatic conditions, how the raw material was collected and stored, and the process used to obtain the oil. Always opt for the best quality oil available.

Know what you're looking, and smelling, for when you shop for oils. Don't be taken in by a sales pitch on the latest, greatest essential oil to hit town. Do your research and go or write to a supplier with a clear knowledge of what you want. Don't be afraid to return an oil if it is not what you wanted, or is of poor quality. I have sent many oils back and told the manufacturer I wouldn't order from them again until they showed an improvement in their quality control. Most companies are anxious to know if a bit of poor oil slipped into their inventory. This problem is most prevalent in some of the larger companies that produce great volume, or where the demand for quantities of an oil is so great that it exceeds the demand for quality.

Find Reputable Suppliers

Knowing the supplier you're buying oils from is the first step. You can shop from the suppliers listed on page 143 with confidence that they are doing their best to supply only the finest, high-quality pure essential oils. Questions as to the origin and purity of an oil are usually met with enthusiasm by someone who is proud of their suppliers. However, I have had shopkeepers assure me that their oils were the best and purest, even after I knew better. So again, buyer beware.

Always look for pure essential oils packaged in full, dark glass bottles, preferably with built-in droppers. These allow you to dispense the oil one drop at a time. (Aromatherapy will, if nothing else, teach you patience!) Some oils are more viscous than others and may take a while to drop out. Some companies have adjusted the size of the dropper or bottle neck accordingly. More often than not, one must be careful. Lavender will drop out much more quickly than sandalwood or vetiver. You can also use a separate glass eyedropper, but do not store it in the bottle because the oil will eventually break down the rubber bulb at the top, which will then contaminate the oil.

Read the label carefully. Look for the term "pure essential oil" and for cautions such as, "Keep out of reach of children," and, "For external use only." These warnings are signs of a responsible company that understands the effects of their product.

Buy in Small Quantities

Whenever possible, buy small bottles. Air in unfilled bottles can accelerate the deterioration of pure essential oils. Keep the bottles cool, dark, and well-filled. I will often transfer small quantities of oils to a smaller bottle if I do not need them for a while.

Avoid Synthetic Scents

I have often wondered how we fell into using synthetics in place of pure essential oils. I believe it has a lot to do with availability. Synthetic scents can be manufactured at a standard cost and rate of production, while we have to rely upon the less-predictable graces of nature for producing pure essential oils.

I have been asked many times for peach, strawberry, apple blossom, or blueberry-scented products. In response, I ask the customer if they know of a way to extract the fragrance oil from

ESSENTIAL OIL SAFETY TIPS

◆ Buy the highest quality essential oils available to you. (I use lesser quality oils to wash my floors, but never my body.)

◆ Dispense by the drop, carefully and count. Record your recipe accurately.

◆ Dilute, dilute, dilute. Very seldom is an oil used "neat" or undiluted.

◆ Use cotton swabs or cotton buds to apply pure essential oils. Using the hands and fingers may eventually contaminate the bottle. Dropper top bottles easily dispense a drop at a time, making it less likely that you will use too much essential oil or accidentally have a spill.

◆ Be careful where you set your essential oil bottles and wipe them clean first. Essential oils can mar surfaces, especially plastic ones. Always make sure bottle caps are twisted on securely.

◆ Practice aromatic etiquette. Many scents may be perceived as offensive to others. Use essential oils and perfumes in moderation in public, and check with family members to make sure your precious vapors aren't causing anyone else distress because of allergies, asthma, or just personal preference.

◆ Label everything — for your own convenience and others' safety. Clearly label and put up away from children any potentially harmful substances. Labeling is a great chance to be creative, too.

these plants. When they reply "no," I assure them that no one else has either, and explain the difference between pure essential oils and synthetic aromatic chemicals.

If you like a certain synthetic scent, fine; use it to scent carpet or to perfume a room spray. Just keep in mind that pure essential oils have qualities and benefits that go beyond the scent. Peach potpourri with aqua-colored wood chips doesn't hold the same magic as a sachet of freshly dried lavender, mint, and rosemary. When squeezed, this sachet releases the pure essential oils from the tiny holding cells in the leaves and flowers. Deeply inhaling synthetic peach potpourri is just not the same and doesn't have the same benefits as inhaling the sweet, deep essential scents of lavender, mint, and rosemary.

I've found from selling my own products at the local farmer's market that consumers are often confused about what they are buying because they've seen so many synthetic concoctions. For instance, my small bottles of freshly made body oils— to which I often add a few herbs or flower buds as well as essential oils — resemble the bottled oils sold just for decoration. Many of those contain artificial, dyed, or decayed flowers and questionable base oils. Their quality doesn't compare to the pure ones I make myself. I must often remind clients that the oils I make are meant to be used, not just admired. It's all part of the educational process.

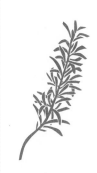

PRECAUTIONS AND CAUTIONS

Working with pure essential oils can be rewarding in many ways. However, it can also be dangerous if certain precautions and cautions aren't observed. Remember that everyone is different and will react to individual essential oils in varying manners. The following simple precautions can make your experiences much more pleasant.

Keep Away from Eyes

Never use essential oils too near the eyes. Keep your hands away from the face, genitals, and mucous membranes when they have been in contact with oils. Always wash your hands before and after working with oils. I wear eye protection when pouring essential oils, and recommend it for you as well. If you do get some oil in the eye, wipe it with a cotton bud that has been moistened with sweet almond oil. Water will just disperse and spread the oil.

Keep Out of the Reach of Children

Pure essential oils can be toxic if ingested in large amounts, and harmful to the skin and eyes if improperly spilled or undiluted.

Children have no place playing with oils unless properly supervised and cautioned.

The use of essential oils on babies is debatable. Some sources say yes, some no. I would not use them on an infant without proper supervision and direction, such as reading *Aromatherapy for Pregnancy and Childbirth* by Margaret Fawcett (see Appendix), attending classes or workshops on the subject, or by visiting a qualified aromatherapist or doctor with experience in this area. I have seen success with using oils on children as young as two years old, and have successfully employed them with my own daughter, Christina, over the years. Lightly scented baths often helped her unwind, right up to today, her first in high school. Evening foot massages have proven relaxing for her many a night.

Children's reactions to pure essential oils vary greatly. Christina had strong positive or negative feelings about oils and strong scents in general. Children, just like adults, take time to adjust to new things including new scents. Let their noses be their guides. Ask them which scents they like and why. The olfactory anchors you create today can span a lifetime.

> **SUNBURN WARNING**
>
> Avoid exposing skin to direct sunlight within six hours of applying citrus oils such as bergamot, lemon, and orange oils. These oils contain components that may cause reddening and blistering or darkening of the skin when exposed to sunlight.

Practice Caution During Pregnancy

There are conflicting opinions on the uses of essential oils during pregnancy. I have heard that absolutely no essential oils should be used in pregnancy, but I also have books detailing just how much you can use. I would advise extreme caution, especially in the first trimester. Many oils can stimulate the uterus, which may be great as birth approaches, but not at two months into the pregnancy.

I have attended births where pure essential oils were used along with jasmine absolute with marvelous results. If you are interested in this use, I advise working with a doctor, midwife, or aromatherapist who specializes in this area. I have heard reports of a reduction in stretch marks when a combination of pure essential oils and very high-quality carrier oils were used faithfully on the skin after the first trimester.

For External Use Only

Pure essential oils are meant for external use only. There are those who practice internal use, but they are doctors or professionals trained in the practice of Medicinal Aromatherapy, primarily in Europe. Using pure essential oils internally would require a great amount of training and testing before it became acceptable in America. I do not suggest that anyone use them internally for any reason.

Avoid Sun Exposure

Some essential oils, including bergamot and other citrus oils, such as lemon and orange, may increase the skin's sensitivity to the sun. The citrus oils can also increase the skin pigmentation in some people. If not properly blended and applied unevenly, darkening and skin irritation could result. According to *Principals of Holistic Skin Therapy With Herbal Essences,* by Dietrich Gumbel, the skin generally has a good reception to citrus oils when properly diluted, applied, and not exposed to direct sunlight. You can purchase bergamot with the bergaptene (the component of the oil that can lead to increased pigmentation of the skin) removed.

BEWARE OF MEDICINAL CLAIMS

I always advise CAUTION regarding healing and medicinal claims made by some when referring to the powers of pure essential oils. ALWAYS consult qualified help when deciding whether to use oils for something other than simple home use. Be sure to consult your doctor before changing any medications or healing practices.

Lemongrass, a fast-growing grass often used in culinary arts, and spice oils such as cinnamon and clove have an irritant effect when used directly upon the skin, due to some of the key chemical constitutes they contain. I saw one client who had a very strong reaction to too much lemongrass (4 ml) she added to a bath. Her skin became red and inflamed, causing her a lot of discomfort. This was alleviated by washing well with soap, showering, and treating her skin with soothing oil mixed with a small amount of lavender, and Roman chamomile.

Remember the Oils Are Concentrated

Pure essential oils and absolutes are very concentrated. Many pounds of herbs, flowers, resins, or fruits are used to produce small amounts of oils. Only small amounts of oil are needed to gain results. "Less is best" is what I tell my work-study students and clients. Many people think that if two drops of an oil will help them feel better, then five or six drops will lead to greater relaxation or stimulation — not so! Using too much essential oil can sometimes have a boomerang effect and aggravate, rather than sooth, symptoms. Essential oils can be expensive, and using less is smart in a financial sense as well.

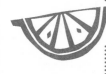

Use Them Diluted

Pure essential oils are almost always used in dilution. Very seldom are they used "neat," meaning undiluted, or straight. Lavender is one oil I feel confident using neat. Tea tree, sandalwood, patchouli, jasmine, and rose absolute have never given me a problem neat. I dab sweet lavender neat on small cuts, scrapes, burns, bumps, and insect bites.

Most other essential oils I use in a dilution of sweet almond oil (see page 65 for exact proportions) or some other base or carrier oil such as grapeseed, apricot kernel, or jojoba (which is actually a liquid wax). For a less oily blend, you can add the oils to a high-quality, unscented cream or lotion base.

Essential oils can also be diluted into shampoos, hair rinses, spring water, alcohol, gels, lotions, and creams. When added to shampoos and rinses, the oils enhance the natural beauty of hair. When added to alcohol, they become elegant perfumes. Another application method is to dilute the oil in a bowl of warm water and use with a compress, or dilute it in a carrier oil or cream that can then be used to massage or condition the skin. Some people suggest diluting oils in milk or cream before adding to a bath, but I just add them directly to the water and stir well. Some people actually prefer the smell of diluted essential oils over the intense smell of the concentrated oil.

Beware of Heat Sources

Keep a keen eye on any heat source you employ to release the scent of essential oils. Candles, simmer pots, and lightbulb rings can catch fire if not properly attended. Forgo using these methods when you are ill or very sleepy. A diffuser on a timer will serve you much better — and keep you safer. Oils on cotton or a small cloth work well when you're tired as well.

LEARNING HOW TO USE ESSENTIAL OILS

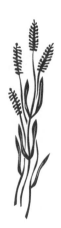

You may be eager and ready to learn about essential oils, but don't know where to begin. Perhaps you will find a mentor who lives close to you who is knowledgeable about essential oils, but chances are good that you may need to tutor yourself (which is why you bought this book!). I am self-taught on this subject, meaning that I have arranged my personal education on my own, taking workshops or classes whenever possible. I want to assure you that it is very possible — and enjoyable — to explore and learn about the world of essential oils on your own, or informally with a group of friends.

Beginning Guidelines

I often conduct introductory workshops for people beginning their educations in this area. Following are some questions I present as guidelines for them to learn more about individual pure essential oils on their own. These questions continue to prove very valuable in my quest for knowledge; I encourage you to use them as well.

Inhale the particular pure essential oil you're exploring and answer the following questions about it.

◆ How do you feel when you smell this aroma?
◆ What do you think this aroma would be beneficial in healing?

- Where on your body would you like to put this oil, if anywhere?
- Which part of the plant do you think this oil comes from?
- How does this essential oil affect you? Close your eyes, inhale deeply, then record how this experience made you feel emotionally, or what you saw as a result.
- Does this essential oil remind you of anything or any place? Make a list of these associations.
- What would you like to blend this oil with?
- Which part of the earth do you think this oil comes from?
- Is this oil masculine or feminine to you, or both?
- Is this essence hot or cold?
- List several words that best describe this aroma.

Go to your books and study guides to learn as much as possible about this particular oil. Then answer the following questions to the best of your ability. Throughout your exploration, remember to enjoy this process of learning about nature's bounty.

- What is the essential oil's name?
- What is its botanical name?
- What is its country of origin?
- Name a few chemical constituents of this essential oil.
- What is the odor intensity of this oil?
- What is the suggested dilution? In which base oils?
- Are there similar oils? Which ones?
- What does this oil blend best with?
- What are the traditional uses for this oil?
- What is the safety data on this oil?
- How can you incorporate it into your lifestyle?

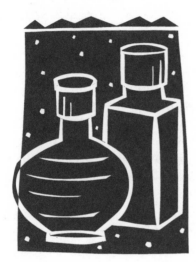

The Properties
and Applications
of Pure
Essential Oils

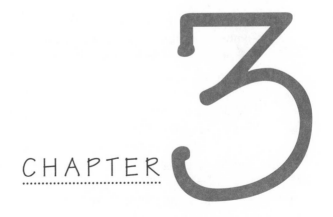

CHAPTER 3

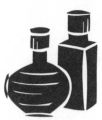

The application of pure essential oils in your life can bring about significant benefit and change when properly employed. Researchers in Europe and America have been studying these precious substances for many years. Long before the term aromatherapy became popular, doctors in France were using essential oils to treat those wounded in wars when medical supplies ran short. Dr. Jean Valnet, M.D. addresses the medicinal uses as well as the antiseptic powers of pure essential oils in his book, *The Practice of Aromatherapy, Holistic Health and the Essential Oils of Flowers and Herbs* (see Appendix). I encourage you to take the time to research the individual essential oils you want to incorporate into your life on your own, as well as checking references by those who have found success in their use. There are several aromatherapy journals available that detail case histories and research. Most are from England, and well worth the price of a subscription. The people submitting these findings have first-hand knowledge and their personal experiences are invaluable to those just beginning their aromatic endeavors (see Appendix, page 144).

MOST COMMONLY USED PURE ESSENTIAL OILS

The following pure essential oils are the ones I tend to use the most. They are also ones I have found my clients and customers seem to use and ask for often. This list is only a sampler of essential oils, absolutes, and oleoresins that are available worldwide today. Most of them are usually easy to obtain and aren't too cost prohibitive to use. Rose and jasmine are expensive, but are usually used in diluted form and purchased in small amounts. If you have a friend who is also interested in using essential oils, you might go in together to buy a bottle of an essence or absolute that is cost-prohibitive to buy on your own. All of the following essential oils have a broad and diverse variety of uses, and most blend together quite well.

BERGAMOT *(Citrus bergamia)*

Nature: The scent of bergamot is delightful, fresh, uplifting, and clean. It stands on its own, or blends well with most other oils. To me, it is a citrus/floral scent. This is a nice addition to personal scents for both men and women.

Benefits: Bergamot is balancing, regenerating, and a necessary essential in every household. This oil seems to have the power to help lift melancholia and depression.

Suggested Uses/Blending: I personally blend this oil with patchouli, lavender, and rose absolute for an all-purpose blend that I use on every inch of my body. I dab this blend neat on little spots or bumps. I also like to bathe in it with sea salt.

Caution: Exposure to the sun can result in a darkening of the skin to which this oil has been applied. I put this to the test a few summers ago by applying neat bergamot on my thumb while I was gardening. Sure enough, that thumb got much darker than the rest of my hand. The darkening of the pigmentation lasted well into the next spring! It was strange being a gardener with a brown thumb. It reminded me of the time I burned my hand badly with a hot glue gun and treated just part of the burn with lavender and vitamin E — once healed, this area didn't even have a scar.

These kinds of experiments have thoroughly convinced me of the powers of pure essential oils.

CLARY SAGE *(Salvia sclarea)*

Nature: Clary sage is a most interesting essential oil. It has become an important part of many of my blends and a favorite herb in the garden. The whorls of flowers are so perfect and beautiful that it seems perfect that they produce a unique essential oil. I love to pass clary sage in the garden, my skirt often rubbing against the leaves and absorbing the oils, only to have them waft up to me later as I sit in the sun.

Benefits: Clary sage has been found to be anti-depressant, anti-anxiety, uplifting, antispasmodic, anti-inflammatory, aphrodisiac, an aid to deeper sleep, and a benefit to the skin and hair care.

Suggested Uses: Clary sage has a place in many body-care products, especially those for hair and skin. I favor it in a hair oil and as a relaxing, regulating addition to shampoos and conditioners. Its antidepressant properties provide an extra bonus in my beauty routine.

As a woman, I would not be without clary sage oil. Its distinct scent has helped me through premenstrual days with grace and ease, as it will through menopause, as well.

Clary sage is effective for men also, and I have known men who love its interesting aroma.

Caution: Some caution must be observed with dear clary as she can get quite out of hand if used too often in too high a dilution. There have been reports of intoxication with clary sage and it is advised never to mix its use with the consumption of alcoholic beverages. Clary is also best avoided in the first months of pregnancy. Use caution when driving after exposure to clary sage. I reserve it for those relaxing times when I can simply rest after its use.

SUGGESTED RECIPES FOR CLARY SAGE

To enhance shampoo or conditioner: Add 1 to 2 drops to ½ ounce of shampoo or conditioner.

For premenstrual symptoms: Blend 3 to 6 drops with 1 to 2 drops of rose otto and 3 to 5 drops of lavender and add to a tub full of warm bathwater.

EUCALYPTUS (*Eucalyptus globulus*)

Nature: Eucalyptus is probably the best-known pure essential oil. Its clean, healing scent reminds many people of some type of medicine. I am often told this oil smells like Vicks VapoRub, a popular chest rub salve. I reply, "No, Vicks smells like eucalyptus." There are many types of eucalyptus, including a lemon one, *Eucalyptus citriodora.*

Benefits: Eucalyptus is an effective insect repellant, and can benefit the skin by acting as an antidote to bites and stings. It also has been found to help relieve neuralgia and muscular aches and pains. I have included eucalyptus in antirheumatic massage oils and chest rubs.

Eucalyptus is believed to be balancing, antiseptic, antidiabetic, antiviral, decongestant, expectorant, insect repellant, fever-reducing, and disinfectant. It has been found effective in cases of asthma. (**Caution:** some asthma is triggered by strong odors.)

Suggested Uses: Eucalyptus has a place in every household. Its antiseptic properties have made it a staple in cases of infectious diseases and epidemics. Its opening powers make it invaluable in fighting sinus and chest congestion. I always burn it in a simmer pot when there is illness in the house to protect anyone who stops by, and to purify and clear the air.

Eucalyptus is a very important ingredient in my world-famous, super-duper, extra-powerful Sniffy Bag™. These little bags were first blended for my daughter when she was quite young and had a bit of a running nose or congestion. She was a breast-fed child, so I would slip the bag into my blouse so she could inhale and nurse comfortably. At night, I would slip one into her pillow and she would wake clear and refreshed.

The Sniffy Bag™ lasts indefinitely if stored in a glass jar when not in use. It can always be rejuvenated with the blend of pure essential oils that are part of its contents which are, of course, called Sniffy Oil™. This oil is a must in cough, cold, congestion, and bronchial remedies. It may, however, antidote homeopathic remedies so you should choose one type of treatment or the other. This has always been a dilemma for me; I must consider each case individually to discern which is most needed. Store eucalyptus well away from any homeopathic remedies.

MAKE YOUR OWN SNIFFY BAG AND OIL

You can create your own sniffy bag by combining equal parts of crushed eucalyptus, peppermint, coltsfoot, and comfrey herbs. The peppermint, coltsfoot, and comfrey are easily grown in a household garden. The eucalyptus can be obtained from a health food store or herb supplier. If you live in a year-round warm climate, you may be able to grow the eucalyptus. I saw lovely large trees while touring herb businesses in California.

To make your own sniffy oil to add to the sniffy bag, combine five parts eucalyptus oil to one part peppermint oil. Combine the sniffy bag herbs first, then add the oil, and mix thoroughly. Put approximately ½ ounce of this mixture in a clean odd sock, knot the end, place it to the nose, and inhale. To store your sniffy bag, place it in a glass, airtight jar to keep the volatile essential oils intact. If you forget to seal it in a jar, simply pour the sniffy bag contents into a bowl, add 8 to 10 drops of sniffy oil, and return it to a new clean odd sock or a small cloth bag.

For a sniffy bath, add 6 to 8 drops of sniffy oil blend directly to the bathwater, or toss in a sniffy bag. This is great to do whenever you feel a cold coming on.

GRAPEFRUIT *(Citris paradisi)*

Nature: Grapefruit is bright, uplifting, clean, and euphoric. It is also cleansing, clearing, and stimulating to the lymphatic system.

Benefits: Grapefruit is believed to help balance the appetite, and has been found useful in treating obesity. It has also been effective in helping to balance the emotions, and has gained high marks from aromatherapists in aiding mood swings. I have personally found it to be very valuable in lifting my spirits. During times of emotional imbalance, grapefruit was there to aid me when all the medical community offered was prescription drugs which weren't the answer for me. Along with juniper, grapefruit is toning to the skin. It is believed to help rid the body of cellulite by cleansing away toxins. It has also been found useful in relieving water retention, congested skin, nervous exhaustion, and stress.

Suggested Uses: I employ grapefruit in baths, massage oils, and skin care. It is the ingredient in my "skinny bath," (see recipe on page 93). The scent is so fresh that I often use it to start a gray, cloudy day when it's often hard to get up and carry on. It seems impossible to stay depressed any length of time with sunny grapefruit as an ally. It is a wonderful citrus note in a personal essence, and I like to put a citrine stone in the bottle to mix it.

Blending: Grapefruit blends well with most oils and adds that light, refreshing note found in summer colognes.

SUGGESTED RECIPES FOR GRAPEFRUIT OIL

For uplifting the spirits: Place a cloth with a few drops of grapefruit oil on the warm clothes dryer in the basement or laundry room and let its uplifting essence waft throughout the house.

For jet lag: Blend 10 drops each of grapefruit, bergamot, and lavender oils in 1 dram (4 ml) of base oil. Rub it into the hands and inhale as needed. Or, add 2 drops of each of the above-mentioned oils undiluted or neat to a bath. I found this blend highly effective in lifting my mood when I arrived in England exhausted from many hours of travel and while trying to adjust to different time zones.

JASMINE ABSOLUTE *(Jasminum officinale)*

Nature: Jasmine, sweet jasmine is one scent nearly everyone loves. It is deep, sweet, floral, and rich. Real jasmine, like rose, is beyond comparison to the imitation fragrances that fill shop shelves.

Benefits: Jasmine is believed to be antidepressant, warming, anti-anxiety, beneficial to the skin and scalp, aphrodisiac, emotionally balancing, soothing, antiseptic, and sedative. Jasmine absolute has been found effective in cases of impotence, frigidity, lethargy, fear, and lack of confidence.

Suggested Uses: A few drops of true jasmine add a heady richness to a personal essence. Added to skin-care products and hair oils, it helps to soothe and moisturize. I love to apply jasmine in my hair and inhale its precious vapors all day long. I apply it by spreading a drop of the pure undiluted absolute across my fingertips and lacing my hair just after washing. A drop of sandalwood is nice as well. This is a wonderful personal treat, especially when I'm on my way to appointments where confidence and emotional balance are a priority. The scent seems to help

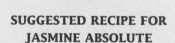

SUGGESTED RECIPE FOR JASMINE ABSOLUTE

For hair care: Combine 2 drops jasmine, 30 drops rosemary, 10 drops lavender, 5 drops clary sage, 3 drops patchouli, and 5 drops sandalwood in a 4-ml amber bottle (label it "Hair Care"). Carry it in your purse and lace 3 drops through your hair with your fingertips, or 3 drops on your hair brush and brush through your hair, as needed, to refresh yourself.

me feel more beautiful and ready to face the day. One added bonus is having complete strangers approach you in public and comment on how wonderful your perfume is.

Long considered an aphrodisiac, jasmine is an important ingredient in my Love Oil. It is uplifting, and seems to exude confidence. Blended with patchouli, rose, sandalwood, and ylang-ylang, jasmine brings out sensuality. It is used in treating impotence and frigidity with great success, because it relaxes the body and soothes the emotions.

Jasmine is the oil of choice for massaging a mother about to give birth, but is too stimulating to be used in early pregnancy. Jasmine massage oil makes a wonderful baby shower gift. It can be very costly, but, like rose, well worth the expense.

To combat depression, try wearing jasmine as a personal essence and let it envelope you throughout the day in a fragrance that has been cherished for centuries by many cultures. Just breathing in the jasmine essence is believed to benefit the respiratory system. Jasmine is a very important part of my personal essence, CKD (see page 125).

Blending: I dilute jasmine in jojoba oil before use, a blend that keeps longer than one made with sweet almond oil. Only a very small amount of jasmine is needed — do not be tempted to use more for a greater effect, since it may actually have an opposite effect when used in too high a dilution. Less is best. Besides, the cost of good true jasmine will limit its use for most folks.

JUNIPER (Juniperus communis)

Nature: Juniper has been a favorite of mine for many years. Its scent seems sacred to me and always clears my mind. I like to add a few drops each of juniper and frankincense to self-igniting charcoal blocks to burn as incense. (**Caution:** Place on a fire- or heat-proof surface. The blocks get glowing red.)

Benefits: I associate the scent of juniper with improved overall health. It is believed to be antiseptic, astringent, diuretic, cleansing, detoxifying, tonic, antispasmodic, parasiticidal, and antirheumatic. Juniper oil has been found useful in cases of edema, skin care, emotional imbalance, diabetes, arthritis, and cleaning.

Juniper has been said to help relieve cellulitis by detoxifying and enabling the body to throw off toxic wastes that accumulate as a result of our contemporary lifestyle. It aids in opening and cleansing the skin, thus enabling it to function more efficiently at eliminating toxins.

Suggested Uses: Juniper is useful in skin-care preparations. It makes an excellent addition to a hair oil, and is wonderful when combined with rosemary and jasmine.

My favorite way to use juniper is in what I call my "skinny bath" (see recipe). Before bathing, I do a salt glow (see recipe on page 92). This helps to eliminate toxins in the body and has helped me shed a few unwanted pounds in short order. Use caution, though, to make sure that the oils and water in your bath are well mixed. I once jumped out of the tub too quickly and some neat juniper oil clung to my hip. The result was an inflamed spot that needed immediate attention. I follow my "skinny bath" up with a massage oil of juniper, grapefruit, and cypress blended in sweet almond oil (see recipe). I like to do these treatments before retiring for the night or as a morning wake-up call, since they can be either relaxing or stimulating, depending upon my state of mind and physical condition.

Juniper has been respected as an antiseptic for centuries. It was employed to clean and disinfect castle and cottage alike. When added to cleaning water, it purifies a home and leaves a clean, woodsy scent. It can be spiritually cleansing as well, and an aid in times when emotions are drained and in need of support.

Juniper also can be used to help rid pets of unwanted vermin, as well as improve their skin.

SUGGESTED RECIPES FOR JUNIPER OIL

For a "skinny bath": Add 5 drops juniper oil and 3 drops grapefruit oil to a warm bath.

For "skinny massage oil": Blend 8 drops juniper oil, 5 drops grapefruit oil, and 5 drops cypress oil in a base of 2 ounces sweet almond oil, or an unscented cream or lotion. Add 2 drops of geranium, lavender, and/or rosemary oils, if desired.

For soothing arthritic limbs: Blend 5 drops juniper oil, 5 drops rosemary oil, 5 drops eucalyptus oil, and 5 drops lavender oil in 2 ounces of sweet almond oil, or your favorite base.

For improving a pet's skin: Add 4 drops directly to bathwater, or blend 2 drops juniper with 2 drops of lavender and mix well into ½ cup powder base (see page 108) to sprinkle on pet as a preventive powder. Another effective formula is 5 drops juniper and 10 drops lavender blended in an 8-ounce spritz bottle of water and used to spray a pet's sleeping quarters or areas they frequent in the home. Add 2 drops of eucalyptus to the spray to help freshen pet's quarters and deter unwanted little guests that may bug your pet.

Caution: Juniper oil should not be used in the first two trimesters of pregnancy or by those who have kidney problems since it may prove too stimulating.

LAVENDER (Lavandula officinalis)
Nature: Lavender's classic floral/herbal scent has been treasured for centuries as a washing herb, and has freshened many a bed linen. Its name evolved from the Latin *lavare*, which means "to wash."

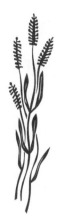

Lavender pure essential oil comes from a number of types of lavender. Its quality and scent may vary — from ones that I think smell like floor wash to ones that smell like heaven. My favorite lavender oil was a small bottle that came through a friend from the Apt region of France. It was wild lavender, or lavender savage, and I truly loved the scent. I still open the bottle years later just to savor the lingering scent.

Benefits: Lavender has been found to be antifungal, antiseptic, antidepressant, calming, normalizing, harmonizing, deodorizing, rejuvenating, anti-inflammatory, anti-bacterial, and is believed to enhance the immune system.

Lavender essential oil has been found effective in cases of stress, insomnia, acne, infection, anxiety, depression, headaches, skin irritations (burns, eczema), and fatigue.

Suggested Uses: Lavender essential oil is what I refer to as my "desert island" oil. It is the one pure essential oil that I am *never* without if I can help it! I have used it when no other was available, and found new uses for it often by trial and error. I have eased busy days into tranquil nights by adding just a drop or two of lavender oil to a tissue, or by packaging the tiny lavender flower buds inside a sachet that can be softly squeezed to release its aromatic oil. I've passed many a summer afternoon making lavender wands. These are stalks of fresh lavender flowers woven with thin satin ribbon into little wands that can be tucked into drawers or luggage.

In the garden, lavender always has a stately green/gray presence. Its flowers, when picked before they open, retain their essence for many years. In my home, I have come across some lavender flowers that have been here for a very long time. Though they are bleached of most of their lovely purple hue, they still smell sweet when crushed. I often just put a handful of lavender buds into a favorite clean odd sock, knot it up, and toss it into a linen drawer. Then I give the sock a squeeze each time I reach in to get a towel, sheet, or washcloth. Lovely lavender smells the same even if devoid of lace, and surely keeps the moths at bay in a much kinder manner than mothballs.

I have often heard stories of memories stirred by the scent of lavender and their association to a loved one. Although the scent of mothballs may conjure up a learned-odor response, the effect is not nearly so sweet, nor nearly so loved, as that of lavender.

Lavender is an essential oil that I count on for small scrapes and insect stings. It is one of the few oils that I feel safe using "neat," or undiluted on my skin. It is a favorite when a blemish pops up at just the wrong time. I simply put a drop on a cotton swab and apply it to the spot. It is very useful in skin care because of its cytophylactic, or cell-protecting and regenerating properties. I have used it successfully on burns received from glue guns or cooking on my woodstove. I keep little bottles on hand during my herb wreath classes in case anyone has a run-in with a blob of hot melted glue.

I often use lavender when traveling on planes to clear the air. However, I knew I had overdone it on a flight to California once when a gentleman seated behind me turned to his wife and asked her if she smelled bug spray! I'm not sure where he got that association, but for me the lavender scent helped me stay relaxed and made the flight much more pleasant.

Blending: Lavender blends with many other essential oils for enhanced healing properties. Some people in France actually use lavender as a base oil. I like to blend lavender with rosewood, bergamot, ylang-ylang, and lemon. It also blends well with rose and jasmine absolute, or sandalwood for an exotic perfume.

SUGGESTED RECIPES FOR LAVENDER OIL

For sunburn relief: 10 drops of lavender oil combined with 4 ounces of water in a spray bottle.

For a peaceful night's sleep: 6 to 8 drops in a simmer pot next to the bed. Be sure to keep an eye on the water level. An aromatic diffuser would also work well for dispensing the oil into the room.

For anxiety or depression: 3 to 5 drops on a tissue you carry with you.

For fresh clothes: Several drops added to the final rinse of the washer, or several drops on a cloth tossed in with the dryer load.

For more enjoyable, refreshing housecleaning: 10 to 20 drops added to 1 gallon (4 litres) of cleaning water to use around the house.

LEMON (Citrus limonum)

Nature: Lemon is a fragrance recognized and loved everywhere. It is a bright, sunny ally to the body, mind, and spirit. The yellow rind yields an essential oil that has numerous uses. Lemon is mentioned consistently through herbal and aromatherapy teachings for toning the skin and helping to balance oily skin. Its use is ancient and far-reaching.

Benefits: Lemon has been found to be antiseptic, astringent, bacteriostatic, and rejuvenating. The essential oil has been found effective in cases of varicose veins, gastric ulcers, skin care, depression, anxiety, and digestive problems.

Suggested Uses: Lemon is great at the start of a meal or a new day. When dining away from home, I always ask for lemon and water. I squeeze the lemon wedge into my water and savor the oil by rubbing my hands together and inhaling the pungent brightness that is lemon. Lemon juice in hot water and a dash of freshly grated ginger root eases the stomach and the sniffles.

Lemon is essential in the home. A sinkful of dishes is made much pleasanter to wash when six to eight drops of lemon essential oil are added to the water — and your hands benefit as much as your nose. Being a gardener, I appreciate the bleaching action of lemon on my nails. Doing the dishes after a day of tending my precious plants is not so bad with uplifting lemon. Once you've squeezed lemons for juice, throw the rinds into a dishpan of sudsy water and use to cut the grease on dishes. I see from the ingredient list on many hand cleaners in auto stores that manufacturers have figured out how well astringent lemon cleans, as well.

I use lemon juice to cleanse small cuts. It stings, but its healing properties are worth a bit of initial discomfort. (Lemon has been found to stimulate the production of white blood cells and aid the body in defense against infections.) Lemon is great for an

CAUTION

The pure essential oil of lemon is much more concentrated than lemon juice, and must be treated with caution and diluted properly before applied to the skin.

As with all citrus oils, avoid direct sun exposure for up to six hours after applying oil on the skin.

uplifting bath or massage when properly diluted. The juice and pure essential oils make good hair rinses, especially for blonds. I often wonder how we've come to use synthetic lemon products when fresh lemon is so available and safe to use.

ORANGE, SWEET *(Citrus aurantium)*

Nature: Sweet orange is a tangy, sunny, bright, uplifting, refreshing scent.

Benefits: Uplifting, skin care, regenerative, antispasmodic, balancing and sedative for some. Sweet orange is an important ingredient in my Uplifting Blend (see recipe).

Suggested Uses: Sweet orange oil is inexpensive and can be used lavishly, if one so chooses. I use it around the house to clean and lighten up the environment. I have also found that a combination of sweet orange, borax, and lavender is an effective carpet treatment for deterring insects, especially fleas.

Children love the scent of fresh, fragrant orange. It is as though someone is sitting next to you, peeling this sweet fruit. Mixed with water, it makes a deodorizing room spray that is effective in dispelling melancholy or depression. A drop or two, no more, is wonderful when combined with vanilla in a bath for children.

Caution: Use caution when exposing skin to sun after oil is applied; some orange oil can make the skin photosensitive. Never leave children to use pure essential oils on their own. They get overly

SUGGESTED RECIPE FOR SWEET ORANGE

As an Uplifting Blend: Combine 20 drops sweet orange, 20 drops lavender, 10 drops grapefruit, 5 drops lime, 5 drops rosemary, and 2 drops jasmine absolute in a 4-ml amber bottle. Spread 3 to 5 drops across your fingertips and lace through your hair. Or add 2 drops to a tissue and inhale, or add 8 drops to a bath. 15 drops blended into 2 ounces of base can enhance a massage and revive a weary spirit. Try adding a few drops of this blend to cleaning water when a task seems particularly daunting.

I reserve this blend for times when life seems to be getting me down and I don't have time to indulge in self-pity. The scent is refreshing and stimulating. Some clients report it relaxes them quite nicely, but I prefer neroli (an essence from the orange flower) for relaxation.

enthusiastic and always use too much! Less is always best when using pure essential oils.

PATCHOULI *(Pogostemon patchouli)*

Nature: Patchouli is not a middle-of-the-road essential oil. It evokes very strong emotional reactions from both men and women. Many associate the scent with that of moist earth, or memories of the hippie generation of the 1960s. Patchouli has enjoyed a history of being considered aphrodisiac.

Traditionally, the scent of patchouli was associated with handmade Indian shawls, which were packed in the leaves of patchouli to ward off insects. My Earth's Essence™ potpourri (see recipe on page 41), which I have made for more than ten years, is a blend of patchouli, sandalwood, and the essential oils and herbs like lavender that have been associated with protecting clothes and linens.

SUGGESTED RECIPE FOR PATCHOULI

As a fortifying blend: Combine 10 drops lavender, 10 drops bergamot, 5 drops patchouli, 2 drops rose absolute in a 4 ml bottle (amounts may be doubled to fill the bottle). Add blend to a bath, or combine a drop of the blend with a few drops of water in your palm and lace through the hair, apply under arms or behind knees to quickly brighten the senses and revive the spirits. Try altering the proportions according to taste.

Benefits: Patchouli is deep and tenuous. Its scent lingers long after other essential oils have faded. It is a good base note in a personal perfume when used sparingly. Patchouli is probably the most abused essential oil when it comes to overuse. Very little is needed to create a long-lasting, lovely, personal essence, massage oil, or skin-care blend. Patchouli adds a depth to blends, and always helps me come down to earth.

Patchouli is believed to be anti-depressant, anti-inflammatory, antiseptic, deodorant, sedative in low doses, and stimulating in high doses. It is also used as a fungicide, cytophylactic, aphrodisiac, and an aid for dry cracked skin conditions.

Suggested Uses: Use patchouli in hair-care blends, personal essences where a deep, earthy note is desired, and baths that are heady, sensuous and good for the skin.

PEPPERMINT *(Menta piperita)*

Nature: Peppermint is a favorite of many people. This herb has touched the masses through flavored breath mints, toothpaste, and sore muscle liniments.

Peppermint is piercing and pungent. Its aromatic coolness is felt as much as smelled. At times, it seems so cold that it is warming, and always must be properly diluted before use. Peppermint oil is strong, sharp, and intrusive, just like its herbal namesake in the garden.

Benefits: Peppermint has been found to be uplifting, rejuvenating, clearing, refreshing, antiseptic, an expectorant, and a mental stimulant. It is also believed to be antiseptic and antispasmodic. The essential oil has been found effective in cases of headaches, congestion, fever, fatigue, sinus headache, migraine, and muscle soreness.

Suggested Uses: Peppermint's cooling effects are appreciated after a day's work outside in the heat. After a peppermint bath you'll feel refreshed and cooler. After emerging from the bath, I like to lie down, put a small fan on low, and fall asleep before the humid weather melts my peppermint aura. My daughter always enjoyed one of these baths when she would come in dusty from a day's play and too tired to fall asleep. Peppermint is too stimulating, however, for a late-night bath. Remember, less is best — you never need much peppermint oil to do a cool job. I often use the fresh or dried herb in place of the oil when only a small amount of essence is needed.

Peppermint tea from the fresh or dried herb has been used for centuries to settle the stomach.

Blending: Peppermint oil is blended with other oils to help relieve congestion,

SUGGESTED RECIPES FOR PEPPERMINT

For a cool, refreshing bath: Add 2 to 4 drops of oil to a tub full of water (do not exceed this amount!).

To relieve congestion: Blend 1 drop peppermint, 2 drops eucalyptus, and 1 drop frankincense with ½ gallon (2 litres) of warm water in a sink or large bowl. Cover the head with a towel, hold over the mixture, relax, and breath deeply.

For sore, overworked muscles: Prepare a massage oil of a base oil with 1 percent peppermint and 1 percent lavender. This is helpful for massaging into the body when you feel a cold or aches of flu coming on.

and is used as an inhalation in warm water.

Caution: Peppermint is believed to cancel the effectiveness of some homeopathic remedies, as does eucalyptus. I recommend using either the homeopathic remedies or the peppermint and eucalyptus. Always store homeopathic remedies separately from pure essential oils.

ROSE *(Rosa gallica), (Rosa damascena), (Rosa centifolia)*

Nature: Once you have inhaled the heavenly scent of rose otto or absolute, you will never again accept an imitation rose fragrance! As I write this, my roses are just in bud, awaiting distillation. This is my favorite time of the year, when the whole yard smells of roses, valerian in full flower, and freshly mown grass.

Benefits: Rose is believed to be an antidepressant, antiseptic, sedative, aphrodisiac, tonic, astringent, and antispasmodic. The oil has been found effective in cases of depression, insomnia, impotence, skin care, nervous tension, feminine complaints, grief, sadness, and low self-esteem.

Rose otto is produced through distillation of the flowers. I don't have enough roses to produce the oil, so I usually opt for producing a high-quality rosewater. This is obtained by distilling roses in a small still, which yields about 32 ounces of pure rosewater. When I am distilling, I'm told that the scent even reaches out to my neighbors several houses away! I wish more people could be exposed to this fragrant process. I don't recommend most of the commercial products labeled rosewater, since they usually contain a synthetic rose fragrance, not true rose oil. You can try making your own rosewater blend by adding two drops rose otto to four ounces spring water. Keep refrigerated because this contains no preservatives.

I do keep the actual rose otto on hand for very special blends that need a bit of extra love. Rose otto oil is solid when cool and warms up to a liquid in seconds when held in the hand. It is expensive and worth every scent cent you spend.

Suggested Uses: Rosewater has been employed as a skin-care agent for centuries. Almost all of my roses go into the production of this precious liquid, and I am very stingy with it. I like to make it last throughout the year. To do this, try storing rosewater in the refrigerator in an amber bottle with a spray top, so you can diffuse it evenly over your face when the day is wearing short and your spirits need gentle reviving.

Rose absolute is obtained when roses are extracted through the enfluerage method. This reddish liquid is just the remedy for emotional imbalances, reminding us to love ourselves. It also draws other love toward us. Try painting a small heart with a dab of rose absolute on the skin over your own heart and rubbing it in. Rose absolute adds a lovely note to a personal essence, especially with a small piece of rose quartz added to the bottom of the bottle.

I add rose otto to a night facial oil as an occasional luxurious ritual. I keep my small bottle of rose otto in a little wooden box my brother gave me. All I need to do is open the lid to inhale its sweet perfume. This oil, with the addition of marjoram, is also helpful in working through grief.

Treat yourself and someone you love to a bottle of rose absolute or otto. Just a little dab can have a great effect on body, mind, and spirit.

Blending: Combining jasmine absolute with rose absolute creates the sweetest bath salts on earth. A few drops of sandalwood added to this blend can turn a bath into a sensual, sweet, calming experience.

ROSE GERANIUM *(Pelargonium graveolens)*

Nature: Rose geranium is another essential oil that people have strong feelings about: They either like it a lot, or they do not! Some change their feelings very suddenly. I have a friend who didn't like rose geranium at all, yet it seemed to be just the oil she needed. I let her take her time adjusting to its scent by suggesting only a small amount at a time. That was five years ago, and now she buys up to four ounces at a time of the best rose geranium I can find — she loves it! When she feels a bit off kilter, she adds six to eight drops of rose geranium to a warm bath. She is on hormone replacement therapy and rose geranium is believed to contain phyto, or plant hormones, that can help the human body's hormone system function properly. Research is being conducted in hormone-rich plants and how they can benefit humans.

The scented geranium plant is lovely to look at, although its flowers are small. The essential oil is obtained from the leaf.

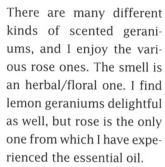

SUGGESTED RECIPE FOR ROSE GERANIUM

As bug repellent: Add 5 drops of rose geranium oil, 1 drop of peppermint oil, and 1 drop of lemongrass oil to 4 ounces of water. Place in a spray bottle and spray clothes before a walk in the woods.

There are many different kinds of scented geraniums, and I enjoy the various rose ones. The smell is an herbal/floral one. I find lemon geraniums delightful as well, but rose is the only one from which I have experienced the essential oil.

Benefits: Rose geranium is believed to be antidepressant, sedative, antiseptic, antidiabetic, uplifting and balancing, and insect repellant. The oil has been found useful in cases of depression, PMS, skin problems, neuralgia, and nervous tension.

Suggested Uses: Rose geranium is added to skin-care products, and can benefit all skin types. It is an excellent bath additive.

Rose geranium oil is a must for many women who need help balancing during those up and down hormonal times.

This oil has a reputation as an insect repellant, and is much more pleasant than some commercial products. Its effectiveness is enhanced when a small amount of peppermint or lemongrass is added. Always wash hands after applying essential oils, and keep hands away from the eyes.

Blending: Rose geranium can quickly overpower a blend. Keep this in mind when adding it to bath, body-care, and perfume oils. It blends well with other oils including lavender, bergamot, clary sage, patchouli, and lemon.

ROSEMARY (Rosmarinus officinalis)

Nature: Rosemary is a beautiful plant to grow and a most necessary essential oil for every home. It is traditionally associated with "remembrance," and was widely used at both weddings and funerals for centuries. Rosemary was burned as an incense in sick rooms to clear the air. I tucked a sprig in my father's casket when he passed away. My beloved kitty is named Rosemary — I could never forget her! Tied on a wedding or gift package, its tradition for remembrance is kept alive. A sprig of the herb, or a drop of the pure essential oil says, "I remember."

Rosemary is also valued for its preservative properties, and was often used in foods during times before refrigeration. I love a sprig or two of fresh rosemary roasted with lamb.

Benefits: Rosemary has been found to be analgesic, antiseptic, circulatory, regulating, antispasmodic, astringent, and a cerebral stimulant. It has been found effective in cases of headache, mental fatigue, cellulite, dandruff, hair loss, and poor memory.

Suggested Uses: Rosemary was one of the first essential oils I got to know. Having long hair, I was aware that the herb rosemary kept it shiny and healthy. I was delighted to discover rosemary pure essential oil as an easier and faster method of highlighting and conditioning my mane. Moreover, its piercing aroma is also known as a stimulant and is indeed a bit of a "wake up call."

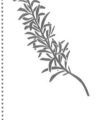

I like to combine rosemary with clary sage, patchouli, and jasmine absolute to make a hair oil to add drop by drop to my wooden brush and comb (see recipe on page 115). The hair is protein in nature and readily absorbs pure essential oils. Their scent stays much longer in the hair than on the skin. This is my favorite place to wear a fragrance or perfume. The rosemary is what one first experiences and as it fades the jasmine, patchouli, and clary sage are left to linger.

Rosemary has been found to also ease stiff, aching, tired, or overworked muscles when used after activity as a massage or bath oil. It has been found to ease rheumatic and arthritic conditions when used in a massage oil. In cleaning water it revives the house *and* the maid! I love rosemary in a bath or shower soap to liven up my morning.

Rosemary essential oil can provide a much needed lift during a long day. Unlike coffee or other stimulants, it doesn't boomerang and end up depleting energy. If I must keep evening appointments it provides a pick-me-up. It is most helpful in a

CAUTION

Rosemary can be irritating to the skin and must be properly diluted before any application to the skin.

Rosemary's sharp aroma has also been employed in inhalations for asthma and bronchitis. However, caution must be used as some prone to asthma are bothered by any scent that is too strong. Caution must also be observed when using rosemary with anyone prone to epilepsy.

simmer pot or diffuser when concentration and alertness are required.

I had some nursing students come to me for help in improving their memory skills prior to their board exams. We combined rosemary with two other cerebral stimulants, lemon and peppermint. They smelled the blend only when they studied and at no other time until the test day. When test day came, the nursing students took scented cotton balls with them, and sniffed their way to a very good score. They happily reported that they felt quite confident that the blend of pure essential oils did the trick to open up locked files in their brains when test nerves began to take over.

ROSEWOOD *(Aniba rosaeodora)*

Nature: Rosewood comes from a tree in the Brazilian rain forests, which is why some people decide to forgo its use. It has a very unique woodsy/floral scent which I love. I find it most useful for the skin and for its balancing effect, which is similar to that of rose geranium. It was once called "Bois de Rose," but isn't found under this name very often today.

Benefits: Rosewood is believed to be balancing, emotionally regenerating, antiseptic, soothing without being sedative, and cell regenerating. It has been found effective in cases of PMS, stress, skin care, headache, depression, nausea, anxiety, and tension.

Suggested Uses: Rosewood reminds me of the wonderful facials I experienced under the skillful hands of Magda Moursi, who has used essential oils in her skin-care salon for many years. If and when you can, indulge yourself in a professional facial. It does wonders for your skin and your soul. When you can't employ a facialist, at least employ pure essential oils in your personal home skin-care routine. Try rosewood in a blend with frankincense and lavender for an every-other-evening facial oil. All three oils are cell regenerating, and produce a wonderful smell just before bedtime.

Rosewood is also nice in hair care: try blending it into a hair oil, or adding a few drops to a hairbrush before use for a refreshing experience.

I am quite fond of adding rosewood to blends for a special note to round them out. It is great in bath products.

SANDALWOOD *(Santalum album)*

Nature: Sandalwood oil didn't impress me when I first experienced its nutty/woody fragrance. Now, years later, I would never be without my deep, sweet, sensuous, spiritually alive sandalwood. Its scent clings like a guardian angel to protect from life's evils. It is soothing to body, mind, and spirit.

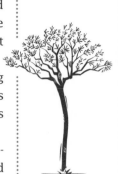

Benefits: Sandalwood is believed to be antiseptic, moisturizing to the skin, antidepressant, expectorant, and aphrodisiac. It has been found effective in cases of dry skin, bronchitis, nervous tension, anxiety, and depression.

Suggested Uses: This ancient scent has perfumed many religious temples throughout time. I have a carved sandalwood bead necklace. I rub the oil into it neat and savor this luscious scent throughout the day. Sandalwood is a great scent for men!

Blending: Sandalwood adds body to a blend, and adds to its staying power. It works particularly well in skin-care blends. In

SUGGESTED RECIPES FOR SANDALWOOD

For bronchitis: Add 6 drops to the water of a simmer pot for soothing relief.

For hair care: Add neat to hair ends to smooth them, provide a sweet sandalwood scent all day long.

For sore throat: Rub the oil neat into the neck area.

For Earth's Essence™ potpourri: In a large glass bowl (don't use wood or plastic that will absorb and retain scent), combine equal parts (such as 1 cup each) of sandalwood chips, patchouli leaves, lavender buds, blue malva, oakmoss, juniper berries, and cinnamon chips or sticks. In a small bowl, combine 2 tablespoons each powdered sandalwood and cinnamon, or any combination of powdered spices you have in your kitchen to equal 2 tablespoons. Add 10 drops of sandalwood oil, 5 drops of patchouli oil, 1 drop of cinnamon oil, 5 drops of lavender oil, 3 drops of juniper oil, and 3 drops of vetiver oil. Make sure the oils are well-distributed by crushing all of the small lumps in the powder.

Add the oiled powder mixture to the herb mixture in the large bowl and mix well. Store in an airtight container (preferably glass) for a minimum of 2 weeks, shaking often to mix the herbs and powder well. Try filling a small cloth bag or odd sock with the mixture and hanging it in your car. When the scent begins to fade, toss the bag up on the dash, turn the heater vent on high for a few minutes, and savor the scent.

a massage oil, sandalwood clings to the skin like a protective film, leaving the recipient with a reminder to relax long after the massage is over. My Earth Essence™ potpourri is redolent of sandalwood, and has been known to last more than ten years (see recipe on previous page).

Caution: Sandalwood takes many years to grow and with the current demand for the oil it has the potential of becoming endangered and expensive. The oil is distilled from the heart wood of the sandalwood tree and it does not grow in very many places in the world. Mysore sandalwood, from a region in India by the same name, is rumored to have some of the finest qualities from which to distill essential oil. You can contact one of the associations listed on page 144 to obtain more information on the possibly endangered status of this fine tree. Luckily, with sandalwood's lingering nature, a very small amount has a lasting effect.

TEA TREE (Melaleuca alternifolia)

Nature: This essential oil is distilled from a tree in Australia, and derives its name from its use as a tea by the aboriginal people. It is a medicinally scented oil, that has a place in every household. Whenever my daughter walks into the house and smells the scent of tea tree she asks, "Who's sick, Mom?" It is one of those desert island oils like lavender that I would never be without.

Tea tree is safe to use neat on the most delicate parts of the body and has been successfully employed during war times when medicines were in short supply. This oil is gaining popularity as an ingredient in personal care products.

Benefits: Tea tree is fungicidal, antiseptic, expectorant, anti-infectious, anti-inflammatory, parasiticide, and antiviral.

Suggested Uses: This a head-to-toe oil that can be used to treat everything from dandruff to athlete's foot. I have experienced a few very nasty spider bites, complete with massive swelling and inflammation. When the medical community offered me little care for these, a combination of tea tree and lavender essential oils applied neat or undiluted to the area helped clear up the bites without scarring.

Yeast infections are very short-lived after antibiotic use of a tampon moistened with ten to fifteen drops of tea tree oil, used daily for seven days. There is *no* other essential oil that I would recommend applying in this manner. Other fungal infections like ringworm and athlete's foot respond well to the tea tree. It also helps heal scrapes, burns, and cuts. I have used it in a simmer pot of water to inhale during times of bronchial congestion.

VANILLA OLEORESIN *(Vanilla planifolia)*, or Absolute
Nature: This easily recognizable orchid scent is a favorite of many folks. The true vanilla oleoresin or absolute is so deep, sweet and wonderful that I include it in my Love Oil!

Vanilla blends great with most other oils, but it will settle to the bottom of a blend and therefore must be shaken well before use. This scent was often used as a perfume during the Depression. I still make vanilla perfume today and use it as a base for many other perfume blends.
Benefits: Vanilla is rarely disliked, in fact it has been shown to be one of the most popular scents known. It tends to remind us of homey feelings like baking cookies and warm feelings. Many find its scent relaxing.
Suggested Uses: Vanilla is a great bath additive, however it tends to sink to the bottom of the tub and has to be well dispersed. I often add it to bath salts instead of directly to the bath water. It also makes a nice addition to massage oils and personal essences in small amounts. These products must be shaken well and often. Vanilla's main aromatherapeutic value is that everyone usually likes it, more than any actual chemical properties it has to help enable us to feel better. Vanilla is one of those scents that once you experience the true scent, the imitations pale in comparison.

YLANG-YLANG *(Cananga odorata)*
Nature: People love to pronounce the name of this pure essential oil. I've heard lang-lang, e-lang-e-lang, and a few other variations. What is important is that the name means "flower of flowers."
Benefits: Ylang-ylang is believed to be antidepressant, aphrodisiac, sedative, calming, euphoric, antiseptic, and hypotensive. It has been found effective in reducing sexual difficulties resulting from anxiety, stress, and depression. The oil has also

been used for cases of rapid heart beat, depression, frigidity, impotence, high blood pressure, and nervous tension.

Suggested Uses: Ylang-ylang is so sweet that it can be overpowering; it must be used in small amounts and high dilutions. I like to use it in baths, relaxing massage oils, skin-care oils, and bath salts. My daughter, who generally finds essential oils too strong for her taste, likes ylang-ylang. When she was younger, I used to put just a drop in her evening bath and she enjoyed it.

My sister found ylang-ylang helpful during her pregnancy when high blood pressure threatened. The scent calmed and relaxed her, which naturally lowered her blood pressure. She added two drops to her humidifier. (Use caution when adding pure essential oils to any thing with plastic internal parts, since too much oil can damage the plastic. However, a few drops twice a day shouldn't hurt.)

I once knew a man who loved this oil so much that he wore it like cologne. I never thought of it as a masculine oil, but he certainly changed my view on that — it works equally well for men and women. How about a candlelight bath for two! With the addition of some soft music and an open mind, wonderful things could result. Try an inhalation, a diffuser, or massage to employ this oil exotically.

Brushing ylang-ylang oil through the hair is a wonderful experience. Remember, only a drop or two is ever needed. Higher concentrations could result in headache or nausea.

Blending: Ylang-ylang can be just the right oil to add a sweet, relaxing note to a blend. I, again, caution about its odor intensity. With ylang-ylang, as with other pure essential oils, one must remember that you can always add more but it is impossible to take them out, so less is best.

Ylang-ylang and lavender baths are one of life's little pleasures. The addition of sandalwood or rose enhances the experience even more.

LESS COMMONLY USED PURE ESSENTIAL OILS

These oils are less commonly used because the general public doesn't have much information about their potential uses. Some of these oils — linden, labdanum, and yarrow — are rare, others are potentially dangerous if improperly used, like hyssop and cinnamon. I include this selected group because I have found beneficial uses for them in my life.

BENZOIN *(Styrax benzoin)*

Nature: This resin has been recognized as a purifier by ancient cultures and is believed to drive away bad energy and evil spirits. Many cultures believed that sweet scents sent heavenward would incur the blessings of their gods. Benzoin has a warm vanilla-like scent. It has been used for centuries in incense and as a preservative in cosmetics. This resinous compound sunk and actually adhered solidly to my bathtub when I used it in a bath to help combat depression.

Benefits: Benzoin has been found to help retain skin elasticity. It is valuable in treating dry cracked skin, and is believed to be antidepressant, anti-inflammatory, antiseptic, an expectorant and sedative.

Suggested Uses: I add benzoin to my Nail Care Oil (see page 111). It works wonderfully to clear up dry ragged cuticles and condition the surrounding skin. Benzoin is excellent as a fixative in a personal essence and very relaxing and soothing in a bath blend or incense.

CINNAMON BARK *(Cinnamomum zeylanicum)*

Nature: Extreme caution must be observed with spicy, hot cinnamon. Be very careful to avoid contact with mucous membranes and eyes. I never use this oil on my body, although others do in a very high dilution. Although true cinnamon essential oil can be caustic to the skin and expensive, it is preferable to the synthetic cinnamon scents available.

Benefits: Cinnamon is best used to scent the environment. A blend of two drops of cinnamon, ten drops of patchouli, and ten drops of lavender mixed with eight ounces of water in a spray bottle makes a superb home air freshener. This formula is antifungal and really makes a musty old basement a nicer place to work. I spray this on my basement stairs and in dark corners that don't get much air circulation or light. The scent lingers and has a spicy, earthy, clean scent. Be careful not to spray on yourself or pets.

A great winter holiday scent is two drops of cinnamon oil blended with ten drops of pine, fir, or juniper oil in water to scent the home for the holidays. Try spraying this blend on carpeting or adding it to a simmer pot. Cinnamon and sweet orange also makes a nice spicy home fragrance.

CEDARWOOD, ATLAS (Cedrus atlantica)

Nature: This is not the cedarwood that reminds us of standing at the pencil sharpener in school or that lines the gerbil cage. The scent is different, not so strong or so pencil-like! The cedar woods of Texas and Virginia do produce a different pure essential oil that is used as insect repellent, is a powerful abortifacient (can cause abortion), and has some aromatherapeutic properties. However, for home use Atlas cedarwood is preferred. It can be soothing, and is used in cosmetics, incense, and household products.

Benefits: Cedarwood atlas is believed to be sedative, an expectorant, antiseptic, astringent, and antiseborrhoeic (balancing to the production of sebum — a secretion from the sweat glands).

Suggested Uses: Add a few drops to a hair care blend. This isn't as overwhelming in scent as other cedar woods, and blends well with sandalwood, juniper, patchouli, jasmine absolute, rosemary, and clary sage — all essential oils that complement a hair blend. I blend it in hair blends for clients with dandruff problems, or hair loss.

Sometimes, I will put cedarwood atlas in a simmer pot to soothe a bronchial problem. It is also fungicidal and is nice in a spray to help control mold and mildew. I add it to my mop water. Try applying some to your tent before you put it away for the season by adding a few drops to water, spray on, and let dry. Patchouli or tea tree blend would work well for this, too.

CYPRESS (Cupressus sempervirens)

Nature: There are several different species of cypress being distilled for an essential oil. This species yields a superior-quality essential oil. Cypress has a pleasant scent that blends well with other essential oils like juniper, bergamot, pine, cedarwood, or lavender. It is a seldom-used essential oil, but very effective when employed. The Tibetan people find cypress purifying and burn it as an incense.

Benefits: Cypress is believed to be astringent, deodorant, styptic, antiseptic, antispasmodic and vasoconstrictive.

Suggested Uses: Cypress is great in a foot bath or powder for sweaty feet. It has been used to make a soothing oil for varicose veins (to be applied, not massaged in). Cypress also helps stem the flow of excessive perspiration in a deodorant blend, and eases heavy mentrual periods when applied as a compress to the abdominal area. I add two drops to a simmer pot to breathe in when I have a cough. Add a few drops in a pet's bath deodorizes and repels fleas.

FRANKINCENSE *(Boswellia carteri)*

Nature: Frankincense has a unique, sweet balsamlike scent. It is a favorite for inhalations and has enjoyed a centuries-old reputation as an incense to cleanse and purify a home or temple. The scent of this fine essential oil is a bonus to its cell-regenerating properties. I love to just smell this precious liquid right from the bottle, and often burn the resin form along with myrrh in my home. Frankincense can be expensive, but the pure essential oil is very much worth the cost and is one I always have on hand.

Benefits: Frankincense is believed to be antiseptic, cytophylactic, anti-inflammatory, and sedative, and an expectorant.

Suggested Uses: I have found frankincense or the "true" incense essential oil to be very valuable as an inhalation for treating bronchitis. The sweet stream swirling up from the simmer pot eases breathing and the spirit.

In a mature-skin blend, frankincense can't be beat. I love to blend it with rose otto, lavender, and sandalwood in a calendula oil base for a facial oil. I also employ frankincense in a body lotion for arms and legs that have been overexposed to the sun. It's pampering, protecting, and comforting.

As a bath oil, frankincense blends well with floral and citrus oils, and deep, long-lasting scented oils like patchouli, sandalwood, or vetiver, a deeply grounding and calming oil distilled from a scented grass. I also add it to a bath with juniper when I feel overburdened. Frankincense is a nice addition to a personal essence blend.

HYSSOP *(Hyssopus officinalis)*

Nature: Opening, tonic, stimulating effect to the respiratory system, antiseptic.

Benefits: This oil isn't in common use, although it is invaluable in pulmonary conditions. I found hyssop most valuable last winter when I had a bout with bronchitis. I added three drops to a simmer pot with six drops each of sandalwood and lavender to help clear my lungs, which were quite tight and congested. After taking a few breaths over the warm simmer pot, I felt relief in my chest. I also added this blend to two ounces of sweet almond oil and used it to massage my chest between inhalations, three times per day. Accompanied by inhalations from a sniffy bag, this treatment helped get me on the road back to health quickly.

Caution: Hyssop should never be used with people prone to epileptic seizures because it has been found powerful enough to trigger a seizure. Hyssop can also be difficult to find, so you may have to find a mail-order source.

LABDANUM *(Cistus ladaniferus)*

Nature: This oil yields from a variety of the rock rose. It was once collected in the wild by scraping it off of the beards of wandering goats grazing in the Grecian Islands. It is not in common use, yet is so unique that I am compelled to include it.

Suggested Uses: I suggest using labdanum oil in an alcohol-based perfume blend as it dissolves and blends better. It adds a deep note to a personal essence and also acts as a fixative to hold the scent. This resinous oil will stain clothing so use caution if adding it to a blend to wear as a personal essence. Labdanum was employed by the ancients as a fumigant to clear the air. The scent is similar to ambergris, a waxy substance secreted from whales, found floating in oceans, and used as a perfume fixative. Ambergris (sometimes referred to as amber oil) and other animal-derived substances such as civet and musk were once popular as perfume ingredients though they are rarely, if ever, found in use or commerce today.

LINDEN BLOSSOM *(Tilia vulgaris)*

Nature: With its sweet, wonderful honeylike fragrance, I love linden in personal essence blends. It is sometimes referred to as lime blossom or lime tree.

Benefits: Linden is a nervine, sedative, and tonic. It seems to elicit a calming influence upon the user and aids in reducing nervous tension. Linden blossom has also been found effective as a soothing and softening agent when added to skin-care products.

MANDARIN *(Citrus nobilis or madurensis)*

Nature: Mandarin is a citrus-scented, sweet, tangy delight. The Italian fruit is suppose to yield a superior essential oil. Mandarin may be photo-toxic and sun exposure must be avoided after use. The scent is refreshing, uplifting, and revitalizing.

Benefits: One of mandarin's greatest benefits is its gentleness. Children love this essential oil and it is gentle enough to be included in their lives. Mandarin is also believed safe to use during pregnancy, so it could be employed by an expectant mother to enhance her household a bit. It is believed to discourage stretch marks when blended with lavender, sandalwood, and frankincense in a good base oil or combination including wheat germ oil. This oil is gentle for the aged too. Even PMS sufferers have found mandarin may ease their distress. It blends well with lavender.

Suggested Uses: A mandarin-scented bath is great when one is feeling blue. Follow it up with a massage with mandarin in the massage oil. Mandarin is a nice part of an uplifting personal essence. Children's rooms and school bags can be freshened with a wipe-down of mandarin in water. An evening massage can be a special treat for a child after homework is done.

Try combining one to two drops of mandarin in two ounces of witch hazel for a refreshing facial or body toner to apply with cotton buds.

PINE *(Pinus sylvestris)*, also called Scots or Norwegian Pine

Nature: There are many pines that yield an essential oil, but not all are useful on aromatherapy. This pine is safer than some cruder distillates. The scent of real pine is so superior to any synthetic creation that I cannot understand why more folks don't use real pine instead of the dreadful imitations. Pine has been recognized as a healing tree ever since humans first discovered that a walk in a pine forest invigorated and decongested. Pine is synonymous with "clean." Its needles and essential oil have been used to disinfect castle and cottage alike.

Benefits: Pine is believed to help clear the mind and clean the environment. It has been employed as an antiviral, antiseptic, expectorant, restorative, and stimulant.

Suggested Uses: I very seldom use pine in a bath or massage oil because it can cause skin irritation. When I do, I use very little and save it for those times when I need a deep refreshing. It also is an essential oil I tend to use more in winter. There is no better scent for the holidays than pine and cinnamon bark, unless it's Siberian fir and cinnamon bark. Add them to a simmer pot or put a few drops of the blend on cotton and tuck them around the house. Both pine and cinnamon can be dermal irritants, so use an eyedropper and wash your hands after handling them. Remember they can mar plastic surfaces. You can also make carpet freshener with these oils to scent the house for a holiday party.

I like pine best when I have the chore of cleaning the house and I am weary. Ten to fifteen drops of pine oil in soapy water can make the task a lot easier and much more beneficial to the housekeeper. The imitation pine cleaners pale in comparison.

ROMAN CHAMOMILE *(Chamaemelum nobile)*

Nature: Roman chamomile is distilled from a certain type of chamomile flower, either Roman or German *(Matricaria recutica).* Roman is clear and sweet whereas German is usually a deep blue/green color and has a much more bitter scent.

Benefits: Chamomile is believed to be analgesic, anti-inflammatory, antispasmodic, and a nerve sedative.

Suggestions for Use: Chamomile oil is a must for headache sufferers. Blend two drops of Roman chamomile oil with five drops of lavender oil in a large bowl of warm water. Take a small cloth towel and barely skim the surface of this mixture with it; apply the warm compress to your aching head. I've found that this treatment in a dark, quiet room works when all else fails. Chamomile oil also works well on sunburn when blended with lavender oil. Taken in tea form, the herb chamomile has a longstanding folk reputation for promoting relaxation and a good night's sleep. It is mild and pleasant to the taste. Be sure to steep the tea for no more than three minutes or it becomes bitter. If this occurs, strain the tea and use it to cleanse your skin or rinse through your hair for added shine. When traveling, I carry a small 2 ml bottle of Roman chamomile in my backpack and inhale deeply of its essence whenever I feel weary. Chamomile herb and oils also make soothing baths. Two drops each of Roman chamomile and lavender oils make a relaxing evening bath. Six drops of this precious essence diffused in a simmer pot of water during times of great stress can transform the mood in the room from harried and stressed to much more tranquil and manageable. This is a good addition to the headache compress treatment for an especially stubborn headache.

Roman chamomile is gentle and effective for children's baths and massage oils when used well diluted. One drop of oil to ½ ounce base is sufficient. The scent is sweet and comforting.

THYME *(Thymus vulgaris)*
Benefits: Thyme is believed to be antiseptic, an expectorant, nervine, antispasmodic, and carminative.
Suggestions for Use: Thyme is a very potent oil and no more than a drop or two is ever needed. Add it to a simmer pot with frankincense and hyssop to clear the air and ease breathing. This pure essential oil was very valuable to me during a bout with bronchitis.

YARROW *(Achillea millefolium)*
Nature: This often hard-to-obtain oil is worth the effort and funds spent in acquiring it. I have distilled this precious herb and found it delightful to watch its azure blue pure essential oil form on the filter paper.
Benefits: Yarrow has similar properties to chamomile. It is believed to be anti-inflammatory, antispasmodic, hypotensive, and carminative.
Suggestions for Use: Use yarrow water like a rosewater for skin. This is the water left from distilling the white yarrow flowers. It is quite wild and strong-smelling, much more like the smell of the flower than that of the pure essential oil. The distillation process is time-consuming and produces small yields. (I garnered approximately ten drops after working for three days and nights gathering armloads of wild yarrow in nearby fields and distilling the flower tops.) You could make a yarrow water similar to the recipe I give for rosewater, by adding two drops yarrow oil to a four-ounce bottle of spring or distilled

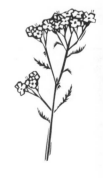

water. Remember to keep this refrigerated and use it as quickly as possible because it has no preservatives. This preparation will smell much sweeter than the by-product yarrow water obtained from the distilling process.

Yarrow has been respected as a healing herb since ancient times. I have used yarrow's anti-inflammatory properties to soothe sunburn by adding five drops of beautiful blue yarrow pure essential oil and five drops of lavender oil to a four-ounce spray bottle of spring water. This mixture can also be added to a cream base to soothe onto the skin. The scent of yarrow oil is very unique and the natural blue hue it adds to skin care products is beautiful.

CAUTION:
ESSENTIAL OILS TO AVOID

There are a number of essential oils that are best to avoid using altogether. These oils can be toxic and have little value for the home enthusiast.

Almond	Pennyroyal
Bitter Birch	Rue
Boldo Leaf	Sage
Calamus	Sassafras
Cassia	Savine
Horseradish	Savory
Lavender Cotton	Southernwood
Mugwort	Tansy
Mustard	Thuja
Onion	Wintergreen
Oregano	Wormseed
Orrisroot	Wormwood

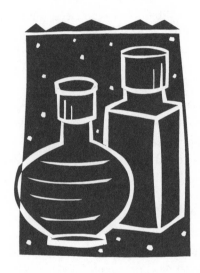

Basic

Blending

Advice

CHAPTER 4

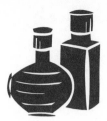

Before you can begin blending and using essential oils, you need to set up a work area. I have a back room of my home set aside for my work area, although my essential oils are stored in the cool, dark basement. I must go up and down the stairs often, but consider this good exercise. You must figure out which area of your home or business will best suit your needs and taste. I prefer the back room because it is away from the hustle and bustle of the main house and is a bit cooler and quieter place, where I can concentrate and work. Good ventilation is important, especially when working for prolonged amounts of time with essential oils. They can become quite overpowering when used in a closed area. I like to run a small fan when working for longer than an hour in an enclosed area. A cool work area is also beneficial. I try to never bottle in direct sunlight, or in a very hot room where the essential oils can quickly evaporate. A flat, even surface that is uncluttered is best. I have had accidental spills that ruined paperwork, labels, and other products.

Easy access to hot water is a must. You'll need to be able to clean your hands and glass equipment such as beakers and bottles with hot soapy water. Some clients have had success cleaning their bottles in a very hot dishwasher — with the pleasant side effect of a lovely smelling home. You will need accessible shelving for storing oils and bases. Arranging the bottles in alphabetical order makes it easier to find what you're looking for quickly and know when it's time to reorder a particular oil.

EQUIPMENT AND SUPPLIES

The equipment and supplies you need to begin experimenting with pure essential oils and absolutes are fairly simple to acquire and assemble.

The most expensive supplies will, of course, be the pure essential oils you choose to experiment with. The bases can also be expensive, depending on which ones you prefer. I suggest trying just a few oils and bases in small quantities to start, and get to know them well. To begin, 4 to 10 ml of pure essential oils and 1 to 4 ounces of base oils are sufficient to experiment with in blending small batches.

The piece of equipment that can be expensive is an aromatic diffuser, averaging from $29 to $100, depending upon the model. Oshadhi/R.J.F. Inc. and Aroma Vera in California offer wonderful lines of diffusers (see Appendix).

For Blending and Storing Oils

Clean dark glass bottles. Collect a variety of sizes from 1 dram (4 ml) to 8 ounces (236 ml). Well-washed old vitamin and tincture bottles work well. This is a good chance to fill those pretty perfume bottles everyone seems to have, but doesn't know what to put in them. Make a perfume to go with the bottle and give it as a gift.

Plastic should only be used as temporary storage for any herb or spice. It is porous enough to allow precious essential oils to penetrate and dissipate into the air. Dark, tightly stoppered or capped, glass bottles are always the ideal storage for herbs and spices and essential oils.

Glass beakers and glass mixing rods. Glass beakers with milliliter measurements are helpful for measuring oils and blends to proper proportions. The lips on the beakers make pouring much easier. I was given my set by a faithful work-study student who worked as a chemist. These are available through biological and chemist supply businesses, which are often found in college towns. Medical supply houses also carry beakers, as well as droppers for measuring pure essential oils. Pharmacies often have bottles and droppers available or a pharmacist may be able to refer you to a source. Bottle companies often have large minimum orders and aren't useful for the home blender. Frontier Cooperative Herbs (see Appendix) offers bottles and droppers in any quantity and a variety of sizes. They also sell a 4-ounce amber spray bottle that is perfect for making personal spray blends or perfumes. Aromaland (see Appendix) also offers good-quality dark amber glass bottles, dropper top bottles, eyedroppers, and aroma lamps. I have had success finding out-of-state suppliers in phone books available in my local library.

Base oils. You will need sweet almond, jojoba, and grapeseed oils for diluting pure essential oils before use.

As I said earlier, 1 to 4 ounces is a good quantity to have on hand to start. I use an average of 8 ounces of sweet almond oil in a month for after-shower rubs, hair oil treatments, bath oils, and my personal massage oils. The amounts I use of other base oils such as jojoba, evening primrose, calendula, apricot kernel, or grapeseed depends on the products I'm producing.

Base oils are available in quantities from 1 ounce to usually 16 ounces in health food stores, co-ops, and even in some grocery stores. I personally prefer to order them from a reputable supplier rather than chance buying a bottle off a store shelf that has gone rancid. Often I will ask the proprietor how long the oil has been on the shelf, and don't hesitate to return a rancid oil. Rancid base oils are commonly found on store shelves, and are identifiable by their off smell. Most base oils have only a light or barely any scent. When a base oil is rancid, the off-smell can overpower the scent of the essential oil added to it, and should not be used. I try to use all base oils within three to six months of purchase.

I add 1 tablespoon of wheat germ oil to every 2 ounces of massage or body oil I make that requires an extended shelf life (more than three months). I also add 10 drops of pure vitamin E (approximately three punctured capsules) for every 2 ounces of base. I very seldom make up blends in advance unless they are to be put on a store shelf or sold at a craft show. I inform my customers that these are to be used as soon as possible and to smell them closely before using if they have been left longer than six months.

Wash items such as massage table sheets, towels, and robes or clothes that come in contact with base oils as soon as possible in very hot soapy water. Buy only what you can use in the near future to avoid using rancid oils.

Sea salt. This is a great base for bath salts. It's also a very economical way to experience one of the precious, costly essential oils since you only need to add a drop or two of oil to a couple cups (approximately 500 ml) of sea salt. I like to mix both coarse and fine grinds. I purchase 5-pound bags of both coarse and fine grinds and blend them in equal parts myself. To make salt glow, only fine grind should be used.

Sea salt is soothing to soak in and looks lovely with small amounts of herbs or flowers added along with the pure essential oils and absolutes. Just make sure the salt is well dissolved in the bath water or you will end up sitting on uncomfortable sharp little lumps. Remember to keep those precious crystals well stoppered to prevent the volatile essential oils and absolutes from escaping into the environment and reducing the potency and effects of the bath salts. Also, salt naturally absorbs moisture so keeping the salts well-sealed prevents this and keeps the mixture from becoming lumpy.

Labels. You need to label every bottle with the ingredients, date of creation, and directions for use. Here's a chance to use your creativity — handmade labels greatly enhance an essential oil collection. For many years, I hand rubber-stamped all of the labels on my products. I created scenes with the sun, butterflies, bees, trees, clouds, stars, moons, flowers, and little animals — and palm trees and dolphins for the citrus oil blends!

The computer opens up all kinds of new possibilities. With the right software, the possibilities are endless.

Stickers add a nice accent to a bottle of essential oil. Victorian motifs with flowers, ferns, lovely ladies, and gardens look great against a dark amber glass bottle. It's fun to search for special stickers that fit the person or occasion for which the oil is being made.

A special handwritten label makes the bottle of blended oils more personal. I like to use gold, silver, or white paint pens to label a special bottle. Just be sure to use ink that won't smear if it comes into contact with the oils. Petroleum-based inks tend to run.

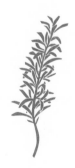

Glass eyedroppers. The rubber tops of these will eventually break down from contact with the pure essential oils. To avoid this, try to collect pure essential oils with dropper top bottles; otherwise, do your best to keep the oil off of the rubber bulb of the glass eyedropper.

For Diffusing Oils

Spray bottles. Collect a variety of sizes from 4 ounces to 16 ounces. These come in handy for everything from spritzing rosewater upon your face to clearing the air in a pet's area. Spray bottles, when well shaken, will propel pure essential oils and water over the body, home, or vehicle. If reusing one of these, make sure it is positively clean and does not contain residue of a toxic substance. I often buy new ones for healing blends I'm planning to spray on the body, and reuse old ones for home cleaning or car care blends.

Diffuser. Aromatic diffusers contain a little glass nebulizer attached to an air pump, much like an aquarium motor. Working without heat, the pump on this electronic device blends air and pure essential oils and sprays a fine mist out into the room. I have seen and tried many prototypes of these little machines, yet rarely use one. One innovative colleague sent me a battery-operated diffuser with an attachment for my belt. I can't imagine needing oils around me that much! The rare times I do use a diffuser are when I need to get a large amount of oils into the air but do not want to heat them, such as when I'm sleeping or not available to keep an eye on the candle and simmer pot. I know people who swear by diffusers and wouldn't be without one. They can be expensive to buy and operate, depending on the pure essential oils one chooses to use. Many of the diffusers I tried actually were damaged by undiluted oils. The oils marred the plastic surfaces and the tubing had to be replaced. Some of the newer models have corrected this problem.

Use caution in choosing a place to set a diffuser. You don't want essential oil mist landing on valuable furniture surfaces it might mar. One advantage of diffusers is that they can be put on a timer. I once played around with making an aromatic alarm clock of rosemary and lemon timed to come on shortly before I had to rise. It was fun, although I am naturally quite time-sensitive and rarely need or use an alarm clock. Not everyone is so lucky. A "diffuser alarm" might be useful if you're a slow riser.

Simmer pot. Lately, these have become very popular gifts accompanied by a bag of simmering potpourri. They are available in most housewares departments of retail stores, and most craft shops. Prices range from $1 for a candle-heated model in the dollar store, up to $15 for an electric model, depending on the size. The simmer pot works by heating water containing essential oils, which are then diffused into the air. I fill the pot with water, then add the desired essential oils, but you must keep an eye on the water level. I have never had one get to the boiling point, but you must use caution to be sure the pot doesn't burn dry! The electric models can be put on a timer.

Simmer pots work well out of doors to drive away unwanted bugs, or in the house when someone has been ill. Because the oils added to a simmer pot or an aromatic diffuser are undiluted, the effects are a bit stronger than oils first added to a base and then applied directly to the skin.

Aroma lamp. These are like simmer pots — minus the water. The pure essential oils are added directly to a warming area and diffused. These can be very elaborate in their designs. These are heated either with a candle or electrically and must be used with caution.

Lightbulb rings. I personally don't use lightbulb rings very often and have seen them catch fire if too much oil was placed on a hot light bulb. They are meant to be placed on a cold bulb, and filled before the light is turned on. I have had difficulty keeping them on the lamp or fitting them between the lamp and the shade. I also had problems with them arriving broken and/or cracked from suppliers so check yours carefully before purchase.

If you choose to use a lightbulb ring, I recommend a ceramic glazed one, rather than the floppy asbestos types. Unglazed ones simply absorb the essential oil, making it difficult to change scents. Rings with a small indentation for holding the oils work better.

Homemade diffusing equipment. If you don't want to invest in any special equipment to start with, you can diffuse essential oils right from your stove. I often add a few drops of pure essential oil to the pan of water I keep on my woodstove all winter. I have also scented a room using an old saucepan on top of the kitchen stove. Another place I have added small amounts of essential oils (ten drops) is the humidifier on my furnace. When sickness threatens members of my household, I add eucalyptus, which works wonderfully to clear the air. Be cautious about using too much essential oil because it could cause damage to internal plastic parts. I reserve this practice for times when it's most necessary, not more than two to three times a winter.

Aroma jewelry. This has become quite popular recently, although I have collected aroma jewelry for more than ten years. My collection includes several necklaces with compartments where pure essential oils can be added, and a pair of earrings with a place to add a few drops of oil. My favorite piece is a cherished gift called a posy pin. This is a small glass vase on a stick pin that can be filled with water so that small flowers and herbs can then be placed in it. I love to fill it with Johnny-jump up, lily-of-the-valley, miniature roses, spearmint, violets, thyme, lavender, chamomile flowers, and soapwort. This little treasure keeps the flowers fresh all day long and, when placed on my lapel, enables me to enjoy their scent wherever I go. Sometimes I also pin it on a hat.

CARRIER OR BASE OILS

Carrier or base oils are the substances that pure essential oils are diluted into for making various preparations, including bath, body, facial, and massage products.

You may choose from a variety of bases, depending on individual needs and preferences. Bases like sweet almond, grapeseed, apricot kernel, avocado, or jojoba (which is actually liquid wax) are oily to the touch. You may also choose to use a cream or gel base. I use them all, depending on the type of skin care or treatment I'm making. Base oils like evening primrose, avocado, hazelnut, rosehip, and calendula can be expensive and are usually purchased and used in small amounts for special blends. I only buy 2 ounces at a time of these. The more common — and less expensive — base oils include sweet almond, grapeseed, and apricot kernel. I often purchase these by as much as a gallon.

Select a base that is as high a quality as your pure essential oils. There is no sense in putting fine oils into a synthetic or mineral oil base. Most essential oil companies carry a variety of bases, or you may choose to experiment with making your own. Many herbal skin-care books have recipes for making your own lotions and creams from natural, pure ingredients (See Appendix). Aloe vera gel can also be used when a cream or oil base isn't appropriate.

Following are some of the base ingredients you may want to have on hand for experimentation.

Apricot kernel oil. Full of vitamins and minerals, this oily base is good for skin-care products for all types of skin. It is especially useful on sensitive and aging skin. I refer to this as mature skin — which includes any skin that is more than 20 years old.

Avocado oil. This is nice as 10 percent of a facial oil. It is beneficial to all skins and contains vitamins and fatty acids.

Grapeseed oil. This oily base is much lighter to the touch than most others. It makes a nice massage oil alone, or combined with sweet almond oil. I like to use it for massaging the back because my hands seem to glide over a larger area easier. It is less viscous than other bases. The best grapeseed oil I ever obtained was fresh from a winery. Its green hue can be detected even in amber bottles.

Jojoba oil. This liquid wax solidifies when allowed to cool. It is an excellent base for personal essences because it doesn't "go off," or become rancid as quickly as some of the others. I use jojoba to extend costly essential oils such as rose, jasmine, sandalwood, and linden. A 10 percent dilution works well. I always list this dilution on my products so clients know the essential oil has been cut. Diluting in jojoba oil is a good avenue for allowing people to experience an oil at a lower cost than buying it undiluted.

Jojoba is nourishing to the skin and hair. I use ⅓ part jojoba oil in hair oils.

Sweet almond oil. Great base for massage, bath, body, and skin-care products. Sweet almond oil is scentless and nourishing to the skin. It relieves dry skin and may be used by itself, unscented, just to condition the skin. I like to apply it after a shower to my still-damp skin. It emulsifies with the water and blends in nicely. The addition of pure essential oils can make the almond oil a key part of an individual skin-care regime. I also combine it with jojoba oil for a hair oil treatment.

Wheat germ oil. Added in a 10 percent ratio to a skin-care product, this yellow oil helps extend the product's shelf life and benefits the skin with its high vitamin, mineral, and protein content.

Other bases. Essential oils may also be added to readymade products such as shampoo, conditioner, skin lotion, powder, dish soap, cleaning bases, as well as to water (for household sprays), alcohol (for perfumes), and sea salt.

GUIDELINES FOR MAKING YOUR OWN BLENDS

When working with a readymade product such as those listed above, start by adding very small amounts of essential oil to the base — only a drop or two per application — until you find a combination you like. Keep a pencil and pad of paper handy to record your experiments, successes, and failures. The best way to learn is to just start blending a little bit at a time. Abide by all cautions on working with essential oils (see pages 15–19) and let your nose, knowledge, and intuition be your guide. Picking up a few really good books on herbs and natural beauty will help too.

You will find guidelines on mixing and blending your own personal herbal and aromatic products at home in natural beauty books, herbals, and aromatherapy books. Look for books with an easy-to-understand format and that require ingredients that can be easily obtained. To identify useful books, ask friends if they have a tried and true favorite book. Reviews in holistic or herbal publications like the magazine, *The Herb Companion* (see Appendix) may also be very helpful.

Another good way to experiment is with a group of friends. Have a day when you get together with friends and make an herbal facial steam, mask, and aromatherapy hair oil. Once you've made your products, trade massages and do a natural manicure and pedicure. These are life's little pleasures and a lot of fun to share, as well as beneficial to your health and beauty.

When blending, it's best to make up small batches that are fresh each time. Most of the bases you're blending the oils with aren't meant to have a long shelf life and contain none, or only a small amount of, natural preservative. Be sure to label what

BODY OIL GIFT PACKAGING

Small bottles of fresh body and bath oils make great gifts. Begin with small (2 ounce) clear glass bottles. (A wide-mouth bottle makes it much easier to remove any spent plant material after the oil is used.) Fill each bottle with a base oil blend (including grapeseed and sweet almond), then add pure essential oils and a few nice dried flowers and herbs from the garden. Like all natural products, these bottles aren't meant to have a long shelf life; they should be used within four weeks.

Try mixing a variety of blends — I like to create a relaxing blend, an uplifting blend, a mature skin blend, a blend of patchouli, lavender, and rose absolute, and a plain lavender one. The oils I like using for these blends include lavender, rosewood, frankincense, rose absolute, patchouli, sweet orange, and clary sage. Vitamin E and wheatgerm oils are nice additions to some blends. For herbs and buds, I suggest rosebuds, lavender sprigs, calendula petals, rose hips, and California bay leaves.

Finish off the bottle with a nice label noting that the oil can be used as a floating bath oil, an after shower or bath moisturizing oil, or as a massage oil, and tie it with a ribbon around the neck of the bottle. It's a good idea also to include a note of caution about avoiding direct sunlight if the blend includes citrus oils like bergamot, sweet orange, and lemon. These are best for evening or indoor use.

you have added and the date. Before using, always make sure that your products are well mixed and shaken so the pure essential oils are evenly distributed.

SOLUTIONS AND DILUTIONS

Solutions refer to the bases that one uses to blend the pure essential oils in, and the final product outcome. Dilutions refer to how much pure essential oil is incorporated into the solution. The solutions and dilutions you choose depend on individual needs and desired strength of the finished product. For instance, I would use a very small amount of pure essential oil in a cream or oil for the face, whereas a larger amount can be used in a cream for the less delicate skin of the arms or legs. A spray intended as a facial toner would have a much smaller concentration of pure essential oils than one intended to be used as a lingering perfume. This is why proper labeling is so very important!

One of the keys to using essential oils successfully is discovering what solution each oil is best dissolved in, and what dilution works best for your needs. This part of working with essential oils can get very exacting and mathematical, which is why this is the part that I am least enchanted with when it comes to using pure essential oils. If you have a propensity for math and calculating, you may enjoy this part. However, mathematical skills are not critical to success, and once you're quite familiar with the process, you can skip the math and begin to use your trained nose and intu-

---

USEFUL EQUIVALENCY MEASUREMENTS TO KNOW

◆ ½ fluid ounce = approximately 15 ml
◆ 1 percent solution = 5 drops essential oil in 4 teaspoons (20 ml) carrier oil
◆ 1 gram (a weight measurement) is approximately equal to 1 ml (a volume measurement)
◆ 1 gram or 1 ml equals approximately 20 drops of essence

SUGGESTED DILUTION FORMULAS

◆ 2 to 5 drops pure essential oil to 1 teaspoon carrier (1 teaspoon = 5 ml)
◆ 6 to 15 drops pure essential oil to 1 tablespoon carrier (1 tablespoon = 15 ml)

ition. But it's best to measure carefully and proceed cautiously when beginning.

I recommend beginning your dilution experimenting with just a few oils. If you buy too many different oils to start, it is very likely you won't be able to use all of them before they deteriorate. As you know, pure essential oils can be costly, so use them wisely. Work with one oil at a time, and get to know each well. Once you've experienced results with these first oils, you're ready to buy more and expand your repertoire.

Measuring Dilutions

The measuring system used for essential oils can be confusing. Some books give dilution measurements in milliliters while others measure in fluid ounces. One simple way to be prepared to use either measuring system is to have measuring devices marked in both milliliters and ounces on hand (these can be found at a biological supply house).

It would be nice to be able to stick with one system of measurement, however most people don't have a milliliter measuring device and many companies sell in ounces and others in milliliters. In the United States, most companies sell products by the ounce, although there is a trend toward converting to milliliters so European recipes measured primarily in milliliters are compatible. For the novice, the best way to start is to measure pure essential oils by the drop. Base oils may be measured either in ounces or in milliliters. I have switched to milliliter bottles in my business to try to avoid confusion. Until aromatherapy practices become more standardized worldwide, measuring systems will be very individual. Measuring in teaspoons and tablespoons is an easy system for the home essential oil user to implement. I very seldom use them because I'm usually blending larger quantities.

Dilution measurements are sometimes given in percentages, such as a "1 percent solution." This means that the essential oil constitutes approximately 1 percent of the total liquid amount. Solutions of 1 to 3 percent are most common in mixing essential oils. A 1 percent solution contains approximately 5 drops of essential oil to 4 teaspoons (20 ml) of carrier (or base) oil. 4 teaspoons (20 ml) of oil is usually sufficient for a full body massage. A very mild blend can be made from 1 drop pure essential oil to 2 teaspoons (10 ml) carrier oil.

Basic Dilution Formulas

The best way to proceed in developing a dilution is drop by drop. Start with 1 teaspoon to ½ ounce (5 ml to 15 ml) of carrier so that you make small amounts at a time. Here are some tried and true formulas to begin with until you have the time and skill to develop your own.

HAIR CLEANSING RINSE
Carrier: 2 cups (500 ml) cider vinegar
Essential oil: Up to 10 drops of pure essential oils of your choice. (Juniper, rosemary, rose geranium, clary sage, lavender, lemon, patchouli, or sandalwood work well.)
Dilute: 1 tablespoon (15 ml) of vinegar/essential oil mixture in 2 cups (500 ml) of water.
Use: Rinse through wet hair after shampooing to rid hair of residue build-up. Vinegar rinses may be drying if used everyday, so it is best to restrict their use to two times a week.

HAIR CONDITIONER
Carrier: 1 teaspoon (5 ml) store-bought conditioner of your choice plus 1 teaspoon (5 ml) cider vinegar
Essential oil: 1 drop patchouli and 2 drops rose geranium
Dilution: 2 cups (500 ml) warm water
Use: Rinse diluted mixture through freshly washed hair and rinse. This leaves hair tangle-free, shiny, and smelling earthy and fresh. After rinsing with this mixture and putting my damp hair up while I work, I enjoy letting it down in the evening and brushing out the sweet smell. Try using other essential oil combinations as well.

SHAMPOO
Carrier: One 12–15-ounce bottle of shampoo (unscented is preferable)
Essential oil: 10–15 drops of clary sage, jasmine absolute, juniper, lemon, lavender, rosemary, rosewood, or sandalwood oils, or any combination of these oils.

The following formulas can be made with carrier and essential oils of your choice.

AROMATHERAPY BATH
Carrier: Tub of warm water
Essential oil: 6 to 8 drops
Use: Add oils just prior to entering the tub and mix well. Dilute with ¼ cup milk or cream, or 1 tablespoon carrier oil, if desired.

CARPET FRESHENER
Carrier: 2 cups (500 ml) pure borax
Essential oil: Up to 25 drops
Use: Mix well. Test for staining before applying to large area.

DISHWASHING FORMULA
Carrier: Sink full of dishwashing water and soap
Essential oil: 6 to 10 drops

FACIAL OIL
Carrier: ½ ounce (15 ml) carrier oil
Essential oil: 6 drops
Use: Apply 5 drops of the blend to the face every other night for two weeks.

FRAGRANT BATH SALTS
Carrier: 2 cups (500 ml) sea salt
Essential oil: 10 to 15 drops (no cinnamon oil)

FRAGRANT BODY LOTION
Carrier: 8-ounce bottle of plain unscented non-mineral-oil-based lotion
Essential oil: 20 to 30 drops (no cinnamon oil)

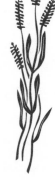

HAND AND SHOWER LIQUID SOAP
Carrier: 4 ounces (118 ml) liquid castile soap
Essential oil: 15 to 25 drops
Use: This soap works great on a loofah sponge, and can help deter the bacteria that builds up on loofah when left damp. Also works well on a small nail brush.

HOUSE CLEANING WATER
Carrier: 2 gallons (8 litres) warm water
Essential Oil: 10 to 25 drops (I like to add Murphy's oil soap to the water as well, according to the manufacturer's directions and depending on the difficulty of the cleaning job.)

INSECT REPELLENT SPRAY
Carrier: 4 ounces (118 ml) water in spray bottle
Essential oil: 5 to 10 drops
Use: Shake as you spray. Don't spray around face and eyes.

MASSAGE, BATH, OR BODY OIL
Carrier: 2 ounces (60 ml) carrier oil
Essential oil: 25 drops (reduce proportionally to make smaller batches)

PERSONAL PERFUME
Carrier: ½ ounce (15 ml) alcohol or jojoba oil
Essential oil: 10 to 15 drops

ROOM FRESHENER
Carrier: 16 ounces (500 ml) water in spray bottle
Essential oil: 20 to 30 drops
Use: Spritz this on furniture, drapes, carpets, and car interior. I also spray this around the damp shower to deter mildew growth. It smells better than most commercial products.

ROOM FRESHENER/INHALER
Carrier: Water in simmer pot
Essential oil: 6 to 10 drops

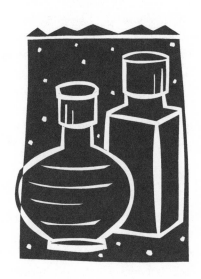

Recipes

for

Home Aroma

CHAPTER

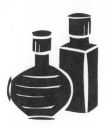

Cleaning the house isn't most people's idea of a good time. However, adding pure essential oils to your cleaning routines can greatly enhance and bring new meaning to this necessary, but often boring, task. Many of the cleaning products available on the market today are full of chemicals. Essential oils offer a natural alternative. While the effects of these oils are not fully researched, I would rather take my chances with their long-term effects than with those of any number of chemical cleansers. Besides, there are known beneficial effects from the oils that can be experienced by your whole family when their use is incorporated into the daily routine. Following are a few suggestions for ways to make essential oils part of your home life.

MAKING CLEANING JOBS MORE PLEASANT

Many folks never consider using pure essential oils in their cleaning routines. As we become increasingly aware as a society of the environmental hazards of chemical additives and cleaners, pure essential oils become a natural alternative to enhance our home and lives in a natural, environmentally friendly way.

Dishwashing

A sink full of dirty dishes is finished up much more quickly in my house when 5 to 7 drops of lemon essential oil is added to the dishwater and dish soap. The steam from the warm water fills my nostrils with bright, tart, sassy lemon — and doing the dishes suddenly isn't such a dreaded task. My hands benefit from the lemon oil, as well, and it also really does help cut grease on the dishes. Sometimes, I'll just throw spent lemons that I have squeezed for freshly steamed vegetables or to make my favorite lemon water, into the dishwater.

I also keep a bottle of vinegar on the sink and add ½ ounce to the dishwater to help glasses and dishes come out squeaky clean. You could add lemon essential oil directly to vinegar and then add this mixture to the dishwater. I would recommend using 10 drops of lemon for 1 ounce of vinegar. One other option is to add this vinegar/lemon oil mixture (or the lemon oil alone) directly to an average 22-ounce bottle of dishwashing soap. I don't have experience adding pure essential oils to an auto-

matic dishwasher since I *am* the dishwasher in my house. However, here again, I caution you that internal plastic parts could be damaged from consistent use of pure essential oils. Occasional use is probably relatively safe.

I often dilute my dish soap, shampoo, and conditioner with extra water as the bottle becomes empty, and I find that these products work much better diluted. They also last longer, which saves me money. Experiment to find which proportions work best for you.

Washing Floors

Next time you're mopping up the floors, try a combination of Murphy's oil soap and pure essential oils, in a ratio of 20 drops of essential oils to 2 gallons (8 litres) of water. I went out into the garden last night during a light rain. My mop stood forgotten up against the house. I could smell the essential oils I had used still on it as I passed by. Whenever guests enter my home they almost always exclaim, "What smells so good in here?" I usually reply, "What doesn't?" Even the tellers at the local bank often tell me that my deposits smell good and they enjoy having them in their drawer. I smile and thank them, although I certainly do not scent my deposits — it's just an aromatic side-effect for the materials that live with and travel with me to shows and classes.

Freshening Carpets

Carpeting can become sour and hold pet smells and smoking odors. I have always treated my carpets to a homemade carpet freshener. Start with a box of borax, available in the detergent section at the grocery store. (This is the aisle I spend the least amount of time in because of the strong chemical smells and overpowering artificial perfumes that scent all the products.) To 2 cups (500 ml) of borax, add 25 drops of pure essential oil. Make sure the drops of oil are crushed well and evenly distributed in the borax. To apply it to the carpet or rug, try shaking it off of a large spoon or out of a large can with a shaker lid. An old powder bottle works well.

RECOMMENDED OILS FOR POWDERED CARPET FRESHENER

Cinnamon
Lavender
Rosewood
Sweet orange

I have two indoor/outdoor cats, Rosemary and Buddy, and I have never had any problem with fleas on them. I attribute this to the consistent use of the borax mixture on my rugs and carpets. If you go into a pet supply store and ask for a natural flea repellant, they will often suggest products manufactured in Florida that contain sweet orange oil. However, using sweet orange oil directly on an animal is *not* recommended.

SCENTING THE AIR AT HOME

I have found many ways to clear the air and scent my home. An aromatic diffuser, simmer pot with water, aroma lamp, or ceramic lightbulb ring can help diffuse oils into the air (see descriptions on page 59). Just remember to use caution with all devices that heat up. Pure essential oils can be flammable and must be attended at all times! One technique I like that requires no special equipment is to add oils to cotton buds and tuck them under couch cushions and in heating ducts. My dear 82-year-old friend Ollie has been soaking cotton buds in vanilla extract, tying them with a string, and hanging them up around her home and motor home for many years.

Here are more ideas for bringing the scents of essential oils — and the plants from which they originate — into your home.

Use Your Clothes Dryer

I have an electric clothes dryer with a vent that can be positioned to blow into the basement instead of outside. I put an old knee-high nylon over the vent to catch lint, then add 7 to 10 drops of my favorite oils to the nylon. Once I start up the dryer, my home smells great in a very short time. Another technique that works well is to put a cloth with oils on it on top of the warm dryer, the scent is released as the dryer heats up. This works with a gas dryer or one that is vented outside. If you have a built-in humidifier on your furnace, this is another place to occasionally add scent.

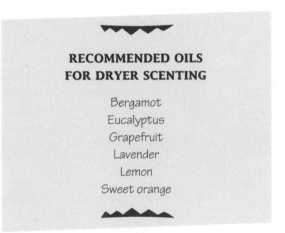

RECOMMENDED OILS FOR DRYER SCENTING

Bergamot
Eucalyptus
Grapefruit
Lavender
Lemon
Sweet orange

The Scents of Drying Flowers

When I open the door to my garden storage shed, the smell from all of the herbs and flowers stored in it is simply wonderful. Don't forget to take advantage of this source of essential oils — the plants themselves. If you're drying fresh flowers and herbs, bring them into your home and enjoy the lovely fragrance they emit while drying. By cultivating your garden outdoors, and then bringing its bounty indoors to dry, you will experience the pleasure of your flowers long after the harvest.

All-Purpose Air Freshener

You can easily make your own air freshener to spray on furniture, floors, and drapes of your home. Add 25 drops of your favorite oil to a 16-ounce (500 ml) spritz bottle full of water and spray. Shake this well as you spritz it around. *Do not spray on the animals or directly on unprotected wood.*

You may choose from quite a few different pure essential oils. (Use caution with patchouli because it may stain lighter

SIMPLE HOLIDAY POTPOURRI

In a large glass bowl or jar, combine the following:

5 parts pine, cedar, fir or what ever greenery you have, cut into small pieces
2 parts small red rosehips (these can often be gathered in the wild) or red rose buds or petals
3 parts dried yarrow flowers
3 parts silver king artemisia (stripped from the stalk)
2 parts whole bay leaves
2 parts rosemary
2 parts small pine cones
2 parts whole spices from the kitchen shelf (including cinnamon, allspice, coriander, cloves, star anise. A package of whole mulling spices without sugar will also work.)
2 parts garden sage, stripped from the stalk
2 parts oak moss
1 part each of the whole resins of frankincense and myrrh, if desired

In a small bowl, make a mixture of powdered spices, proportionate to the amount of potpourri, i.e., for 2 cups potpourri, use 1 teaspoon spice mixture. (If you don't have a lot of spices, cinnamon alone will do.) Add 1 drop of cinnamon bark oil, 5 drops rosemary oil, and 5 drops pine or Siberian fir oil to the spice mixture. One drop of frankincense can also be added, if desired. Make sure the essential oils are well distributed in the spice powder blend. Use a spoon back or a mortar and pestle to crush up the little drops of powdered oil.

Add this mixture to the potpourri.

Seal the finished potpourri to make it airtight, shake well, and let stand for two weeks. Package in nice little boxes tied with raffia, with a whole cinnamon stick and sprig of rosehips and greenery on top.

If desired, you can blend the essential oils in an alcohol base like vodka to create a refresher oil that can be added to the potpourri as needed. You could package a 4 ml bottle of this combination and an eyedropper on top of the potpourri in the box.

fabrics.) My choice is greatly influenced by what season it is and what is going
on in the house. If I am having a meeting requiring
attention and alertness, I
may use rosemary or
lemon. For a romantic inter-
lude, I'll use sandalwood,
lavender, clary sage, ylang-
ylang, and jasmine ab-
solute. If someone in the
house is feeling the first
signs of a cold coming on,
I'll add eucalyptus, thyme,
and lavender or tea tree.

For the Christmas sea-
son, I love to spray the
house with the scents of fir,
pine, cinnamon, pepper-

RECOMMENDED OILS FOR AIR FRESHENER SPRAY

Bergamot
Eucalyptus
Grapefruit
Juniper
Lavender
Lemon
Pine
Rose geranium
Rosemary
Sweet orange
Ylang-ylang

mint, clove, frankincense, myrrh, and juniper. In summer,
lemon, grapefruit, rosemary, lavender, sweet orange, and
patchouli oils scent the rooms. In the spring and fall, I fill my
rooms with bulbs, flowers, fresh and drying herbs, and enjoy
the scents of the flowers themselves.

Creating a Bedroom of Flowers

The bedroom is a wonderful place to introduce the sweet smells
of essential oils. I love to strip my bed, wash the linens in aromatic water, and then line-dry them. For the rinse, simply add
a few drops of essential oils to the final rinse cycle in your
washer. If you're using the clothes dryer, you can place a few
drops on a cloth and add to the dryer.

While the sheets are drying, turn your mattress and spritz
water laced with essential oils into each side of it. If you prefer,
wipe the mattress and bed down with a bowl of water and oils.
After making up the bed, indulge in a fresh herbal bath before
retiring upon sweetly scented dreams — much like people have
done for centuries (minus the washer and dryer!).

Another nice way to freshen a bed is with a pillow sachet. I like to keep a lavender sachet tucked into my pillow to gently scent when lain upon. A friend once gave me a pillow sachet made from an old lovely lace-edged hankie filled with cloves, dried spearmint, and lavender flowers. Tied with a satin bow, it looked every bit the little forgotten treasure that used to be much more common.

MEMORIES OF THE SWEET SMELL OF HOME

Every home and house has an "odor print" — a collection of odors, scents, and smells that we recognize as home. We build these odor prints from the time we're very young, and the memory of them lasts a lifetime. Pure essential oils help keep our homes protected, while lending their sweet scents to our family history. Following are some ideas for building pleasant scent memories for your family. Once you become attuned to this element of the home environment, you will develop more ideas of how to make it pleasant, sweet, and memorable.

Pomanders

I have made pomanders, clove-studded oranges rolled in spices, for many Christmases. Now I have a basket of these spicy treasures ready to set out each year. I know my daughter will never smell the scent of this fruity spice mixture without being transported back home for the holidays.

These aromatic treasures are easy to make and can brighten up a chilly fall or winter evening. Begin by piercing holes in the orange one at a time with a square toothpick and adding a clove to each hole (see Figure 1 on page 78). The square stems of cloves fit nicely into these holes, and not too much juice runs out from the orange. Also, the cloves stay whole and don't break from the pressure of pushing them through the skin without a premade hole. Be sure to make the holes in an arbitrary pattern; if they are all in a row the orange may split on the dotted line.

When the orange is completely covered with whole cloves, roll it in a spice mixture of ground clove, cinnamon, and star anise (see Figure 2). Be sure to cover the whole orange so it doesn't rot. Pass a small crochet hook through the middle of the pomander and pull 1 yard of gold cord or ribbon through it (see Figure 3). Tie off the end and hang the pomander up to sweetly scent the room (see Figure 4). If desired, you can just roll the oranges in the spices or leave them to cure in the bowl of spice mixture.

Note: Some people add a powdered fixative called orris root to the spice blend to give it extra lasting power. I don't add it because of potential allergies associated with its use, and I have found the staying power of my pomanders to be fine. For old pomanders, I simply rinse them off each holiday and re-roll them in the spice mixture. If you have trouble finding powdered star anise the clove and cinnamon mixture alone will do.

Pomanders make priceless gifts and are a nice family tradition to get started. The aroma of orange and spice is comforting and festive. This is a great project for children to work on them while waiting for a holiday meal to be prepared. I take a basket

SUPPLIES FOR MAKING POMANDERS

2 small, thin-skinned oranges
4 ounces whole cloves
Several square toothpicks
½ cup ground cloves
½ cup ground cinnamon
½ cup ground star anise
Small crochet hook
2 yards of gold cord or festive ribbon

MAKING A POMANDER

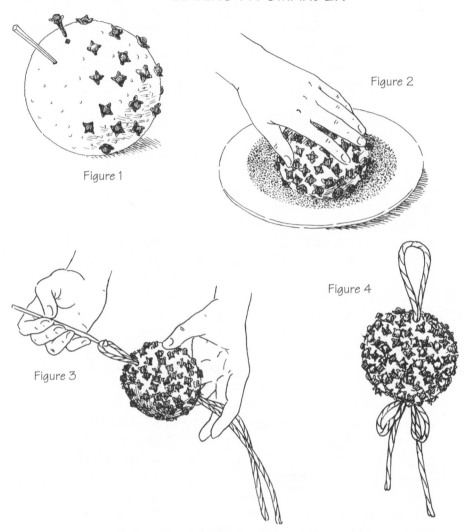

Figure 1

Figure 2

Figure 3

Figure 4

of supplies with me to holiday arts and crafts shows where I'm exhibiting so children can try their hand at making one while their parents shop. Many people have memories of making these in scouts, church camp, or school when they were young. Once I had a group of kindergartners in my daughter's class each finish a pomander in an afternoon. The way I motivated them to finish was by placing the spice mixture in a large shaker can with a sign on it that read "Magic Dust." A six-year-old will go to great lengths to shake a can of magic dust!

The Smells of Cooking with Fresh Herbs

The smells of cooking can turn a house into a home. Adding fresh herbs and spices to that cooking enhances the flavor and the memorableness of a meal. The smell of something cooking often wafts out the kitchen window while I am working in my gardens. My work is speeded along on the savory wind so that I may go in and enjoy my meal. Herbs can be grown in a simple cook's garden outside a kitchen door for easy access, or in pots on a deck or porch. In addition to the basic cooking herbs, a lemon garden is a nice addition, which would include lemon verbena, lemon balm, lemon thyme, lemon basil, and lemon geranium.

Memory Potpourri

During a trip to England and France I gathered a small amount of herbs or flowers from each person and place I visited. I would wear some of these in my posy pin on my lapel during the day and put them in a basket to dry at night. By the conclusion of my trip I had a fine memory potpourri to commemorate my trip. This was a souvenir that money couldn't buy and a memory that will last as long as I stir and savor the deep glass bowl containing my aromatic mile markers.

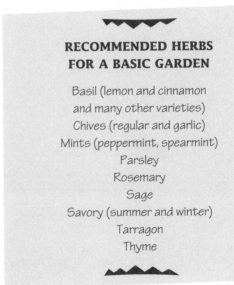

RECOMMENDED HERBS FOR A BASIC GARDEN

Basil (lemon and cinnamon and many other varieties)
Chives (regular and garlic)
Mints (peppermint, spearmint)
Parsley
Rosemary
Sage
Savory (summer and winter)
Tarragon
Thyme

Included in my memory potpourri are: lavender and rose petals from my host's door yard, roses from Paris, mint from a neighbor's door yard, herbs and spices from castles I visited, rosemary from outside a hotel I stayed in, and pine cones from an ancient forest. This smells lovely and the only essential oils in it are the ones contained in the plants themselves, nothing extra was added.

Scent is a wonderful way to remember meaningful life events and experiences. Save all of your flowers from weddings, graduations, proms, funerals, baby showers, bridal showers, or those given to you by a lover or friend to make a memory potpourri that can be shared and savored for years to come.

To make the potpourri, remove the flowers from the stalks and place them in a large bowl (see Figure 1). Mix together small amounts of your favorite spices in a small bowl (for a total of two tablespoons [30 ml] of spices). Add 10 to 20 drops of your favorite pure essential oils to the powdered spices (see Figure 2). Make sure the oils and spices are well blended. Pour this powder mixture along with some whole spices such as cinnamon sticks, star anise, allspice, or coriander over the dried flowers and close in an airtight container for 2 to 3 weeks, shaking the container daily. Open, place in one of your treasured dishes, and enjoy the memories (see Figure 3).

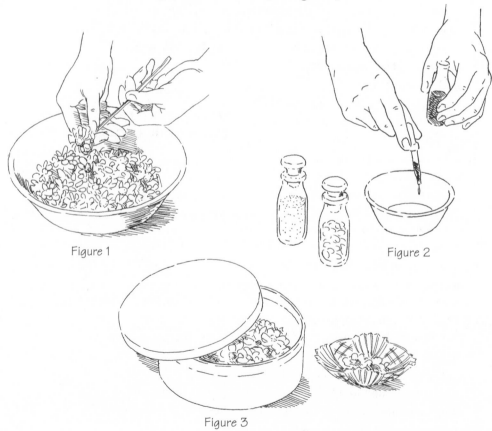

Figure 1

Figure 2

Figure 3

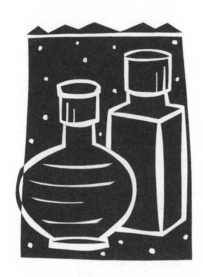

Aromatic

Recipes

for Essential

Beauty

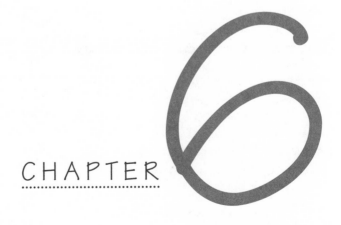

CHAPTER

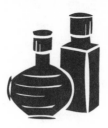

One of the great joys — and benefits — of learning to use essential oils is being able to blend your own natural beauty treatments. Beauty products found on store shelves today often contain a number of additives or preservatives. One of the surefire ways to know that the ingredients in your beauty products are fresh and of the highest quality available is to make them yourself. For centuries women have enhanced their appearance through the use of natural, botanical-based beauty aids.

As anyone knows who has indulged in an occasional facial, massage, or day at a beauty spa, pampering yourself with these treatments can be very beneficial to both mind and body, but they can also be very expensive. Besides, then you've still got to drive home, which can quickly interfere with the relaxation you've just achieved. Creating your own home spa can provide you with quality products at a fraction of the cost you would pay in a department store or salon.

CAUTION ABOUT ADDING ESSENTIAL OILS TO THE BATH

Essential oils should be added to a bath just before you enter the tub. If added to the water while the tub is filling, much of the oils' precious essences goes up in steam and very little is left to be absorbed by the skin. Then you get the benefit of inhaling the scents, but you miss out on the benefits to the skin.

Once you've added the oils, be sure to mix them into the water well. It is very important to avoid direct skin contact with undiluted essential oils that may irritate or cause skin sensitivity. You can also dilute the essential oils in a carrier oil before adding them to the bath or, as some people prefer, in ¼ cup milk or cream.

Remember that less is best. Adding more essential oils will not necessarily help you feel better than a small amount of oils will. These are very concentrated and should be used sparingly and well-diluted. As you become familiar with the oils, their intensity, and your own personal reaction to each of them, then you may feel comfortable experimenting with a larger number of drops of selected oils. But, generally, err on the side of too little rather than too much. Pure essential oils are much more concentrated than the herbs in the leaf or flower state and deserve your respect.

By making your own blends you can enjoy an "oasis" day and then just melt away right in your own home for as long as you want. You can also be sure that it is only selected herbs and pure essential oils — without any synthetic or harmful chemicals — that you're covering yourself with from head to toe. These "self-care days" present a wonderful opportunity to share special times with a few friends as well — making up your own personal blends, trading massages, and taking turns enjoying herb and oil baths, hair oil treatments, and salt glows.

Homemade beauty and health care products also make lovely gifts — and conjuring up creative names and finding attractive containers to package them in can be half the fun of making them. Unscented base creams are available from several sources listed in the Appendix. These are nice for making moisturizers and skin creams when an oil-based skin-care product isn't appropriate.

BATHS

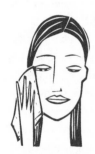

Bathing with pure essential oils is one of life's greatest pleasures. The oils lend their healing powers to the warm bathwater and diffuse aromatic magic all around you. Add your favorite music and a candle glowing nearby and you have a completely wonderful experience.

Bathing enjoys a rich and redolent history. Reviving such a beneficial practice makes good sense. Many folks say they are strictly shower people. If you're one of them, try one of these baths. Or if you're close to a shower-only person, prepare an aromatic bath and let him or her re-evaluate their loyalty.

Many a problem has been soothed away while watching aromatic vapors swirl through candlelight. I have enjoyed deep, profound states of relaxation that enable me to stay balanced in a busy world. I have turned to the tub when all other means to relax have failed. Once I lock that door and start the water running I am in a world of my own. Sore and overworked muscles are soothed enough to allow restful sleep by steeping in a warm tub laced with nature's helpers — pure essential oils and herbs.

On summer mornings, I enjoy bright, stimulating baths of rosemary, lemon, or peppermint before going out to walk at the lake or plant in the garden. Cranky PMS days send me looking for the lavender, clary sage, bergamot, and rose absolute or otto. A morning bath can turn around a day that didn't get off to the best start.

Making Your Own Bath Blends

With a sound knowledge of the necessary precautions for using pure essential oils (see page 15), anyone can have great fun experimenting with bath blends. Experimenting is a necessary part of learning how pure essential oils blend. As you become familiar with each oil and its individual characteristics and odor intensity, blending will become much easier to comprehend. Often you may develop a blend that is actually more potent than the total of its individual components.

MY FAVORITE COMBINATIONS FOR ESSENTIAL OIL BATHS

◆ lavender, ylang-ylang, patchouli, and rose absolute
◆ lemon, juniper, grapefruit, and rosemary
◆ bergamot, rosewood, sandalwood, frankincense, and clary sage
◆ lavender, rose geranium, and patchouli
◆ lavender, rose absolute, and bergamot
◆ sweet orange, vanilla oleoresin, and frankincense

I'm sure you will discover your own favorites as you explore and experiment with these rich natural resources. Be sure to keep a pad of paper and pen in a basket in the bathroom so you can record your favorites. Many of the best ones come together unexpectedly, inspired by the need to balance a particular feeling or day. These are great opportunities to let your nose be your guide.

Maximizing the Effects of the Bath

One of the best ways to prepare your body for bathing is to dry brush the skin with a natural-fiber brush before bathing. This technique, which can be done daily, opens up clogged pores and eliminates dead skin. You simply brush your entire body, except for the face (and breasts for women), for 5 to 20 minutes.

Begin gently, and then work up to a more vigorous brushing, beginning with your hands, then arms, underarms, neck, chest, stomach, back, legs, and feet. Your skin will glow, and be ready to receive the beneficial effects of an aromatic bath.

Following the bath, instead of drying with a towel, try massaging plain unscented sweet almond oil directly into wet skin. The oil mixes with the water and emulsifies into a wonderful skin conditioner that seals in moisture. Essential oils that complement your skin type may be added to the sweet almond oil. A 2 percent dilution works well (see page 64). This blend could also be used as a floating bath oil. Blends of base and essential oils can be used instead of undiluted essential oils in the bath, but the blend is oilier. I prefer using these blends when I am not washing my hair in the same water, since, while good for the hair (see page 113), the base oils leave it looking and feeling oily. Undiluted essential oils don't leave an oily feel because they actually dissipate in the water and evaporate into the air.

WAKE UP BATH I

3 drops rosemary
3 drops lemon
2 drops eucalyptus

For bath: Add oils directly to a tub full of warm water and mix well.
For shampoo or shower soap: Add blend to 1 ounce unscented shampoo or liquid castile soap.
For massage or hair oil: Add blend to 1 ounce base oil.

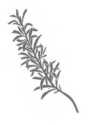

WAKE UP BATH II

3 drops rosemary
2 drops peppermint
3 drops lemon

See directions above.

REFRESHING BATH

3 drops bergamot
2 drops grapefruit
3 drops rosewood

For bath: Add oils directly to a tub full of warm water and mix well.

This blend can provide a boost when you're feeling weary. It's refreshing without being either over-stimulating or sedating.

COLD CARE BATH I

5 drops eucalyptus
2 drops peppermint
2 drops lavender

For bath: Add oils directly to a tub full of warm water and mix well.

As inhalant: Add blend to a simmer pot in a sick room. Be sure to watch the water level.

For massage oil: Add blend to ½ ounce base oil and massage into the chest.

This pungent blend opens the nose and soothes aching muscles. It is effective when a cold is coming on. Before using it, apply to a small patch of skin on the inside of the arm to test for skin sensitivity. Never apply pure essential oils "neat," or undiluted, without testing them first.

COLD CARE BATH II

3 drops frankincense
3 drops hyssop
6 drops eucalyptus

For bath: Add blend directly to a tub full of warm water and mix well.

As inhalant: Add blend to a ceramic simmer pot full of water that has been candle-warmed. Make sure the mixture is not too hot! I like to hold the top part of the simmer pot between my hands and as they are gently warmed I inhale the aromatic vapors, breathe deeply, and relax. I add the oils three times per day, 4 to 6 hours apart.

The blend can also be used as an inhalant in a bathroom sink or large bowl of warm water, with a towel placed around the head to help direct the vapors up the nose. I like to use the simmer pot because I can curl up with it anywhere I am comfortable. The scent is warm and spicy and feels good as you inhale.

As massage oil: Add blend to 1 ounce base oil and massage into chest, arms, neck, and abdomen. The vapors are released by body heat. Take a warm bath with the essential oils and follow with this massage.

If someone else is around who can massage the oils into your back and feet, the road to recovery is usually much shorter. They need not be a certified massage therapist, although a professional massage is always an advantage in most healing processes.

For treatment on the go: If you *must* go to work while suffering from a cold, try what I call travel tissues. Blend the oils and add them to tissues; store these in a bag you can carry all day to inhale as often as possible.

If this blend smells too medicinal to you, add a drop or two of a favorite oil such as ylang-ylang, rose geranium, or jasmine absolute to sweeten it to your taste. I have found that the addition of 1 to 2 drops of chamomile (Roman) or clary sage helps me relax and stay in bed — and resist that urge to get up and work when I obviously need rest!

On hair: I have long hair and will often add the diluted massage oil to it. The heat from my head then diffuses the aromatic vapors all around me — and my hair gets conditioned in the process. I also employ my personal facial oil to keep the skin around my tissue-sore nose from flaking. I believe the antiseptic properties of the oils help protect people I come into contact with from getting my cold as well.

I have found this blend useful when I feel that congested, tight feeling in my chest which often accompanies a cold or flu. Remember that you should always see a doctor for a proper medical diagnosis before pursuing any course of treatment.

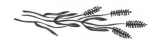

RECIPE FOR MY
PERSONAL FACIAL OIL

Blend 2 drops frankincense, 2 drops rosewood, 2 drops rose otto, and 2 drops lavender in 15 ml base.

As a base, I recommend 2 ml evening primrose, 2 ml calendula, 1 ml wheat germ, 10 ml sweet almond, or any other base of your choice (2 ml is approximately ½ teaspoon; 15 ml is approximately 1 tablespoon). I usually blend this mixture in larger quantities and refill a 15 ml or ½-ounce bottle as needed. This smells heavenly and feels so good on the skin.

PMS BATH

Combination 1

3 drops clary sage

3 drops lavender

2 drops rose absolute or
  otto

Combination 2

2 drops clary sage

3 drops lavender

2 drops chamomile
  (Roman)

2 drops rose geranium

For bath: Add either combination of oils directly to tub full of warm bathwater and mix well.

For bloating: Add oils to ½ ounce base oil and 2 drops of juniper and massage into the abdomen.

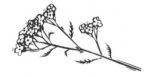

PMS — premenstrual syndrome — can strike fear into the hearts of men, and surely give any woman who has had to deal with it a reason to groan. It's no fun being out of sorts, bloated, and cranky. I've found that personalized herbal formulas and the use of pure essential oils can significantly reduce painful and distressing PMS symptoms such as tears, confusion, angry outbursts, and tender, swollen abdomen and breasts.

RELAXING BATH

5 drops lavender
2 drops ylang-ylang
2 drops rose absolute or
    otto

For bath: Add oils directly to a tub full of warm bathwater and mix well.

For massage: Add to ½ ounce base oil and 2 drops Roman chamomile (optional) and massage over the body before rest. This blend smells wonderful.

BATH OIL GIFT BOTTLES

Make up bath oil blends in larger quantities to divide up and package as gifts in dark glass bottles. You can use either pure, undiluted essential oils or a blend of oils diluted in a base oil to use as a skin softener. For undiluted bath blends, you'll need bottles that hold ½ to 1 ounce; for diluted floating bath blends, purchase 2- to 4-ounce sizes.

Make the gift complete by creating a nice label that clearly states the ingredients, cautions, and number of drops to use (or capfuls in the case of diluted blends). I always include the date the blend was made and my initials, as well. Rubber stamps and colored ink pads offer lots of options for graphics and lettering on your label. If you are making a large quantity of bath blend for shower favors or fundraiser items, you can order decorative address labels by mail with your blend information printed in place of your name and address.

I like to hand make labels from either readymade sticky-backs or paper cards that can be hung from the bottleneck. If you use sticky-back labels, cover them with a protective layer of clear tape once they're on the bottle so they last longer. Paper cards can be paper punched and tied on the bottle with a piece of ribbon. Tie on a glass eyedropper with each bottle, unless you can find bottles with dropper inserts. Eyedroppers come in sizes to fit specific bottles. I use ones that fit 4 ml (1 dram) and 15 ml (approximately ½ ounce) amber bottles.

EXOTIC EVENING BATH (WORTH THE EXPENSE!)

2 drops jasmine absolute
2 drops rose absolute
4 drops sandalwood
2 drops vanilla
2 drops ylang-ylang

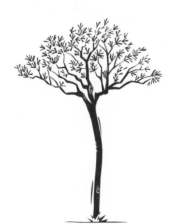

For bath: Add oils directly to a tub full of warm water and mix well. This is a wonderful bath blend for two. Add soft music and candlelight to enhance the experience.

For a sensual massage: Add essential oils to 1 ounce base oil for a sensual massage. The formula can be doubled for two! 3 to 5 drops of lavender may be added for a relaxing touch.

For a warm, exotically-scented massage: Place base oil in a simmer pot and warm slightly, then add the pure essential oils. This blend is sweet, relaxing, and sensual for both men and women.

ANTI-DEPRESSANT BATH

3 drops bergamot
3 drops rosewood
3 drops lavender
2 drops rose otto

For bath: Add oils directly to a tub full of warm water and mix well.

For massage: Add essential oils to ½ ounce base oil and massage over the entire body, especially the heart area. For a full body massage, double the amounts in recipe.

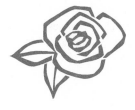

GRIEF BATH

3 drops sweet marjoram
3 drops lavender
3 drops rose absolute
1 drop cypress

For bath: Add oils directly to tub full of warm water and mix well.

For massage: Add essential oils to ½ ounce (15 ml) base oil and massage into the heart area.

EASING GRIEF

Along with the homeopathic remedy Ignatia, the Grief Bath blend has helped me through the deaths of close friends and the endings of difficult, emotionally painful relationships. The Bach Flower Remedy formula Rescue Remedy is another treatment I've found very helpful in easing grief and the shock that often accompanies it.

BATH SALTS

Adding pure essential oils to sea salt makes wonderful bath salts. This method is especially useful when using very expensive oils such as jasmine and rose absolute since it only takes a few drops added to 2 cups (500 ml) of sea salt to make an elegant blend. While 1 or 2 drops of these oils alone doesn't seem like much for enhancing a bath, when mixed thoroughly into sea salt these drops are extended and make for a very pleasant bath. Sea salt detoxifies the body and conditions the water and skin. (It's great for scrubbing the oily film off your tub as well!)

Base oils such as sweet almond, apricot kernel, or grapeseed oil can also be added to the sea salt/essential oil blend to make a salt glow (see following recipe).

SALT GLOW

2 cups (500 ml) sea salt
1 ounce base oil
6–8 drops essential oil or
   absolute

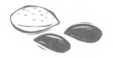

For exfoliating massage and bath: Combine all ingredients in a bowl and mix well with your hands. Make sure to crush the little drops of oil that clump in the salt. Stand nude in a dry bathtub and gently massage the body, starting with the feet. Work your way up, massaging in a circular, clockwise motion. As the oiled salts fall to the base of the tub, pick them up and reuse them until the entire body (except for face and neck) has been massaged. Then fill the tub with warm water and soak your cares away. The skin becomes soft, stimulated, and sweetly scented.

This blend is useful for exfoliating dead skin cells on the body (although it is too harsh for the delicate skin of the face and neck). The skin literally glows after applying and bathing in this blend.

BATH SALTS GIFT JAR

Bath salts make a lovely gift. When properly sealed they can last a long time. To ensure a longer shelf life, do not add base oil to the salts (you can include instructions for doing this just before use on the label). For a very special blend, try adding 1 to 2 drops of jasmine or rose absolute to 2 cups (500 ml) of salt. Add some lavender or clary sage (2 to 4 drops each) to enhance the relaxing powers of a sea salt bath. Find a pretty jar, make a special label, and give this gift to a friend who's experiencing their share of exasperating days.

AROMATIC BATH SALT BLENDS

There are endless combinations of essential oils for bath salts. These are a few favorites that work well. The recipes can be easily doubled to make more.

BATH SALTS COMBINATION #1

3 drops lavender
3 drops grapefruit
2 drops juniper
2 cups (500 ml) sea salt

For relieving cellulite: Make sure the oils are well mixed with the salt to avoid skin irritation. Then take a "skinny bath" in these salts that have been found to help relieve cellulite. Follow up the bath with an application of the oils blended in ½ ounce base oil to particular areas where cellulite is a problem. Cypress oil is a good addition.

These essential oils are known to help cleanse toxins from the body, and the scent is clean and fresh. Drinking a lot of water is also very important when cleansing the body of any impurities, as is maintaining a healthy diet and lifestyle.

BATH SALTS COMBINATION #2

3 drops sandalwood
3 drops patchouli
3 drops lavender
2 cups (500 ml) sea salt

This is an earthy, grounding blend that men tend to especially like.

BATH SALTS COMBINATION #3

3 drops rosewood
3 drops bergamot
2 drops frankincense
2 cups (500 ml) sea salt

This is a balancing, refreshing blend. If desired, add 1 or 2 drops of a citrus oil like lemon, sweet orange, or tangerine to brighten this blend.

SEA SALTS COMBINATION #4

3 drops eucalyptus
2 drops peppermint
2 drops benzoin absolute
  resin
2 drops cypress
2 cups (500 ml) sea salt

For salt glow: If you don't have the time or place to take a full bath, try doing a salt glow on just your feet or hands, then soak them. This is a divine thing to do after you've been working them all day.

This is a great blend to bathe in when a cold is coming on.

AROMATIC GIFT BASKET

Make an aromatic bath basket, including two herbal bath bags (see directions on page 96), a jar of bath salts, and directions for a salt glow. Other items you could include are: a small bottle of liquid castile soap, a loofah or scrub, an assortment of three pure essential oils in 4 ml bottles with eyedroppers, and a small bottle of sweet almond oil (2–4 ounces). Some appropriate essential oils would be: lavender, rosemary, sandalwood, ylang-ylang, rose geranium, grapefruit, clary sage, bergamot, or rosewood.

Line the basket with a fine washcloth or small towel and sprinkle a mixture of dried herbs in the bottom before adding the goodies. Use herbs you've included in the bath bags, or lavender and rose buds for beauty, calendula petals for brightness, or mint leaves for an aromatic and stimulating tone. Let your nose be your guide.

Be sure to label each item and add creative directions for use. Lovely decorator bags work well for gift packaging, too, and can be found in many varieties. This basket of aromatic allies will be a cherished gift.

HERBAL BATHS

Baths with whole herbs and flowers are another enjoyable way to enhance the bathing experience. These bath sachets make most welcome gifts. They are traditional, economical, and ecologically safe. They can be personalized according to the language of flowers, or just according to your own likes. Blends can be made for various skin conditions or just to relax and enjoy. A good herb book can help guide your choices. Remember that herbs have a much lower concentration of essential oils than the pure oils, and they have to be crushed to release them.

It is preferable to store bath herbs as whole as possible to retain the essential oils. The herbs should be well dried, and the bags stored in a glass jar if they are to be kept for any length of time. Dry the bag between baths, and once you're finished bathing with them, put the used herbs in the compost pile.

I am often asked why I tend toward the essential oil world

instead of being an herbalist. I reply that I'm just a lazy herbalist — adding a few drops of pure essential oil to a bath recipe often seems much easier than preparing and working with the herbs themselves. I advise you to try it for yourself, and see what you prefer.

How to Make a Bath Bag

Select any combination of four to five of the suitable bath herbs. Blend in equal parts (see Figure 1).

Select material for making bags. These can be odd socks, knee-high nylons, hand-sewn bags, or pieces of muslin — whatever works best for you (see Figure 2). Cotton washcloths work well filled with herbs and tied with a rubber band and ribbon. These make great party favors or shower gifts. Use dark-colored washcloths as some of the herbs may stain a light-colored fabric. Add a handful of herbs to each bag. (A handful is the one measuring device that I always have near and it never varies! For centuries this was used when nothing else was available. I have even seen old pioneer cookbooks where ingredients are measured in handful, child handful, and doll handful.)

To use the bag of bath herbs, tie it on the water spout while the tub is filling, or toss in like a big tea bag. Scrub yourself with the bag and squeeze it often to release the oils from the herbs.

SUITABLE BATH HERBS

All of these herbs can be easily grown in a home garden or ordered from an herb supplier (see Appendix, page 143).

Calendula
Chamomile
Comfrey
Garden sage
Lavender
Lemongrass
Peppermint
Rosemary
Rose
Spearmint
Thyme
Yarrow

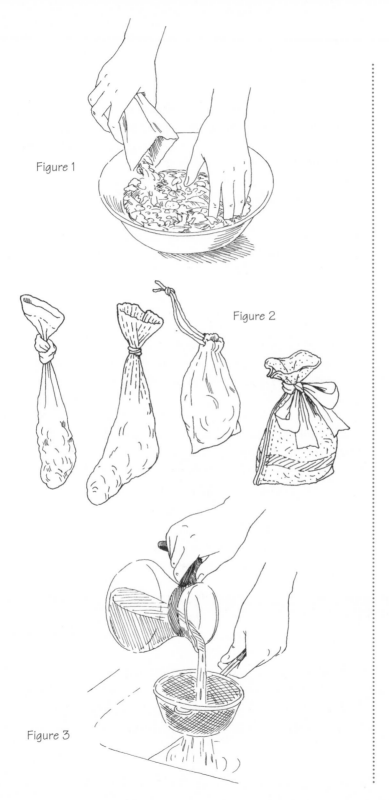

Figure 1

Figure 2

Figure 3

Alternative Methods for Herbal Baths

♦   If you're daring, and have a plumber in the family, you can toss a few handful of herbs directly into the tub. Don't try this, however, if you have temperamental drains. Actually, most of the herbs stick to the bottom of the tub when the water drains out. It's fun to watch the herbs float in the bath, and even more fun to comb the floaties out of your hair when you're done.

♦   Simmer the herbs in 3 quarts (3 litres) of water in a non-aluminum pan; strain the resulting tea into the tub (see Figure 3 on page 97).

CHILDREN'S HERBAL BATHS

Children are always destined for a warm bath. They are also very much in tune to the sense of smell, so combinations of pure essential oils are an effective and fun way of enticing them into the tub.

These recipes are great evening bath blends that help an active child unwind. A follow-up massage can be a great opportunity to spend quality time with a child and a wonderful way to show you care and are there to listen. A parent's caring touch is an oasis in an often challenging world.

CHRISTINA'S CREAMSICLE BATH

2 drops sweet orange
2 drops vanilla oleoresin

For bath: Add essential oils to tub full of warm water and mix well.

This blend was developed as a surprise for my daughter when she was 5 years old and loved to buy creamsicles — orange-coated vanilla ice cream on a stick — from the ice cream vendor. It smells yummy and makes it a bit easier to get a dusty 5-year-old to come in from play.

LEMON DROP BATH

2 drops grapefruit
2 drops lemon

For bath: Add essential oils to tub full of warm water and mix well.

The bright scent of lemon in the house can entice a kid in from the backyard. This blend is especially good at getting a grubby child squeaky clean. Lemon is so cleansing and refreshing.

SLEEP-EASY BATH

2 drops ylang-ylang
3 drops lavender

For bath: Add essential oils to tub full of warm water and mix well.

This is a soothing, relaxing blend that helps ease away a day's stresses and strains. This one seems to help ease some of the emotional lumps and bumps of childhood.

SUMMER'S EVENING BATH

2 drops peppermint
3 drops lavender
2 drops chamomile
(Roman)

For bath: Add essential oils to tub full of warm water and mix well.

For sunburn: Add essential oils and 1 tablespoon (15 ml) apple cider vinegar to a 4-ounce spritz bottle filled with water and spray on sunburn.

For colds: If your child has a cold coming on, try the Cold Care Baths (see page 86). Just make sure the blend is well dispersed in the water! Sitting on the side of the tub while the water is filling, with the door closed, is a good way to inhale the vapors and help relieve congestion.

This blend is especially useful for children suffering from overexposure to the sun. It will soothe the burn and cool the body. After the bath, tuck the children in with a fan set on low and they will soon be fast asleep. Try this one for adults, too!

FOOT BATHS

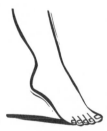

Sometimes there isn't a tub or the time available for a full body bath. This is when an aromatic foot bath is greatly appreciated. We don't often realize just how important our feet are. We stuff them into ill-fitting shoes, stand on them for long hours, and never give them much notice until they are blistered or in pain.

Reflexology is based on the belief that every organ of the body is connected to a reflex point in the foot and other parts of the body. There are points believed to stimulate the digestive, respiratory, lymphatic, circulatory, glandular, reproductive, and nervous systems. Reflexology training is gaining popularity as people search for ways to enhance their preventive powers by keeping the body as a whole in better balance.

Massaging and stimulating these reflexology points by applying finger pressure has beneficial effects on the associated part of the body. It is further believed that the muscles, bones, sinuses, and even the whole body, can derive benefit from this practice. When a certain part of the body is experiencing imbalance this is often reflected by varying degrees of discomfort that is felt when the appropriate reflex point on the foot is stimulated by massage. For further explanation on reflexology and the use of pure essential oils in this practice, refer to the excellent guide contained in *Practical Aromatherapy: How to Use Essential Oils to Restore Vitality*, by Shirley Price. After further investigation, you may well decide to add a bit of foot massage after your aromatic foot bath.

Since she was very young, my daughter Christina has loved having her feet soaked and massaged. She would come to me often and say, "Mom, will you please do my feet?" It became a time for us to talk, relax, and just enjoy each other's company. Give someone you love a coupon book for foot soaks and massages you'll administer at their pleasure. I guarantee this will be a welcome gift! A foot bath is a wonderful treat for everyone — child, adult, and senior citizen.

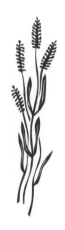

Dish Basin Method

The basic equipment you need for a foot bath is a vessel that is large and deep enough to allow your feet to fit comfortably, and holds enough water to cover the feet up to the ankles. I prefer a plastic dish basin or enamel wash basin because it is deep enough to keep the water from sloshing over the sides when carried or from overflowing when the feet are submerged. I haven't used essential oils in the automatic foot baths that vibrate and massage the feet. My concern would be for the internal plastic parts, if any, that might deteriorate as a result of contact with the oils.

A dish basin is also easy to clean and portable — you can sit in front of the TV, or read and relax on the couch, while soaking tired feet. It's good to keep a kettle of water heating on the stove so you can keep warming up the foot bath as needed. Remember to set a towel next to your soaking area so you have it ready to wrap up those relaxed toes when you're finished.

SPECIAL TREATMENT
FOR SORE OR SWOLLEN FEET

A cold water foot bath is a great treatment for swollen feet or a foot or ankle injury. Keep some ice cubes nearby too for extra soothing.

I use homeopathic arnica gel or ointment to treat any sore overworked muscles or sprains. This works wonders for bruises, swelling, and stiffness caused by physical trauma. Arnica can also be taken internally in the form of homeopathic pellets and or tincture, available in most major health food stores. Arnica montana is an herb that is respected for its healing properties. Although the herb itself isn't taken internally the homeopathic preparation has been found safe and effective. The ointment and gel are used externally on unbroken skin. Arnica gel helped ease the sore feet of this world traveler and I would never leave home without it. Arnica massage oil is also very useful for massaging sore feet or an overworked back. Arnica ointment should be put on last, following an essential oil massage blend.

The art and science of homeopathy, which goes back to the eighteenth century, merits further investigation by anyone interested in holistic healing. The consultation and guidance of a homeopathic physician is recommended for serious conditions.

Begin the bath by washing your feet with pure castile soap and water before putting them into the basin to soak. Essential oils should be added to the basin just prior to immersing your feet. A total of 8 to 10 drops essential oil is enough, and the combinations are endless. I prefer peppermint, rosemary, lemon, patchouli, rose geranium, bergamot, lavender, eucalyptus, tea tree, or clary sage. As with a tub bath, one must make sure the oils are well dispersed in the water before entering the water.

A foot bath can be done at the office, as well. It doesn't take much space to store a dish basin and a few towels. When traveling, blend your foot bath oils ahead of time and carry them with you. In a hotel, the tub method (described in following section) works best.

Tub Method

Another way to take a foot bath is to just sit on the side of the tub on a thick towel and dangle your feet. Wash your feet with castile soap first, drain the tub, then add enough warm water to cover your feet up to the ankles. Add the essential oils after the tub is full, and sit and enjoy inhaling their aromatic vapors while your feet soak in their beneficial effects. More warm water can be easily added as the water cools. This is also a foot bath you can share with a loved one or friend. Children usually enjoy foot baths, as well, and more than one of them can sit on the edge of the tub at once to clean up grubby little toes.

AFTER THE BATH

A foot bath is further enhanced when followed up by a foot massage with a blended oil. This also coats the feet with a protective film of oils. A nail treatment is also a nice accompaniment. (See nail oil recipe on page 111.) Once done, I like to put on warm socks and curl up, most contentedly. What could be easier or more relaxing?

I use the tub method when I've been outside gardening and my feet are covered with earth. Also, after a long day on my feet it's easier and quicker than hauling out the dish basin.

Liquid soap dissolves any oily residue left in the basin or tub.

Foot Bath and Powder Recipes

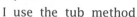

Individual needs and the condition of the feet being bathed should guide you in choosing the most appropriate essential oils. Foot baths are especially helpful in treating tired, aching feet, cases of ingrown nails, foot fungus problems such as athlete's foot or ringworm, injuries, or sprains.

Foot bath blends usually contain 8 to 10 drops of pure essential oils to 2 gal-

CAUTION

Pure essential oils mixed in an oily base before being added to a bath may make the tub surface quite slippery. Watch your step when entering and leaving the tub!

lons (8 litres) water. One cup (250 ml) of Epsom or sea salts can be a nice addition to these foot baths. The essential oils can also be mixed with base oils (see box on page 104) and added to the warm water in this form, or undiluted, which tends to keep the basin or tub from becoming oily.

TIRED TOOTSIES BLEND

3 drops lavender
3 drops rosemary
4 drops lemon

Add oils to 2 gallons (8 litres) warm water and mix well.

This blend comes in handy when I've been on my feet all day at a show and still have things to do at home before I can totally relax. The lavender soothes the feet and the rosemary and lemon refresh, revive, and stimulate circulation.

ATHLETE'S FOOT BATH

4 drops tea tree
4 drops lavender
2 drops sandalwood

Add oils to 2 gallons (8 litres) warm water and mix well.

This combination of pure essentials works wonders for people plagued with chronic athlete's foot problems. Tea tree is anti-fungal, as is lavender. The sandalwood conditions, softens, and soothes sore, cracked feet and toes. Its antiseptic and soothing properties help keep feet safe from secondary problems that can arise from the open cracked skin.

Patchouli could be substituted for sandalwood as a skin regenerator. Patchouli also has fungicidal properties.

FOOT AND HAND MASSAGE OILS

Any of the foot bath blends can be made into foot or hand massage oils by adding essential oils to 1 ounce of base oil. These massage oils may be made up in advance and kept on hand (or foot!) for use when needed. Remember to store them in dark glass bottles and avoid exposure to heat, light, and air.

BURNING FOOT BATH/BLISTER BUSTER

3 drops peppermint
4 drops lavender
3 drops chamomile
(Roman)

Add oils to 2 gallons (8 litres) warm water and mix well.

This is a favorite for worn, weary feet that have been moving all day. I love this one when I have been traveling and my feet are stuffed into shoes and on the move from morning to night. The peppermint cools, and the lavender and chamomile soothe both my feet and my spirit. Arnica gel, ointment, or massage oil is perfect after this bath. If blisters are present, I take my arnica internally and use calendula gel or ointment on my faithful feet. Taking an internal dose of arnica (a homeopathic formula available in most health food stores) during the busy day is also an option to avoid any chance that the peppermint in the footbath may cancel out the effects of homeopathic remedies.

RETURN-TO-EARTH FOOT BATH

3 drops patchouli
3 drops sandalwood
4 drops lavender

Add oils to 2 gallons (8 litres) warm water and mix well.

This deep, rich, earthy scented blend is a perfect foot bath for those times when life leaves us up in the air. These pure essential oils are believed to be relaxing, centering, and calming. The scent of sandalwood has been used in meditation rituals by many cultures. I once had a client tell me that he knew of a culture that believed that the way to heaven was by rubbing sandalwood oil between the toes. Perhaps this could be better called "heaven-on-earth" blend. Juniper can be substituted for patchouli.

Sandalwood pure essential oil is a luxury worth affording. I offer it to clients diluted 10 percent in jojoba oil: 10 drops sandalwood to 100 drops jojoba. A small dram, or 4 ml bottle, is approximately 60–80 drops: 6–8 drops sandalwood to 4 ml jojoba. (If you're making the mixture in the bottle, use 5 drops of sandalwood and 50 drops of jojoba to allow room to mix.)

RECYCLE ME FOOT BATH

3 drops bergamot
3 drops clary sage
4 drops rosewood

Add oils to 2 gallons (8 litres) warm water and mix well.

This is a bath for full days when you must be going strong into the night. Rosewood and bergamot are refreshing and are neither too sedating or stimulating. Clary sage is the pure essential oil that helps soothe away the day's cares and tensions on aromatic vapors.

I like to soak my feet for about 15 minutes, just lay back, relax, and follow with a 15 to 30 minute nap for a complete revival. If you don't have time for a nap, just a quick soak can be reviving in itself.

MY ACHING FEET BATH

3 drops lavender
3 drops eucalyptus
4 drops rosemary

Add oils to 2 gallons (8 litres) warm water and mix well.

This combination is for those occasions when you know you should have brought along more comfortable shoes. This blend is refreshing and soothing. A follow-up application of arnica gel will put you right back on your feet!

FLOWER TOES BATH

3 drops lavender
3 drops ylang-ylang
3 drops rose absolute or
  rose geranium

Add oils to 2 gallons (8 litres) warm water and mix well.

Reserve this blend for those leisurely days when you have time to indulge yourself in an elegant cloud of floral relaxation. Lavender, ylang-ylang, and rose absolute is one of my favorite blends. The rose geranium is a nice addition or substitution for the rose absolute, adding an herbal green note to this blend and helping condition the skin of the feet.

CHILDREN'S FOOT BATH

2 drops sweet orange
2 drops ylang-ylang
2 drops mandarin

Add oils to 2 gallons (8 litres) warm water and mix well.

This is one of those hang-your-feet-over-the-side-of-the-tub and wiggle-your-toes baths. Mandarin pure essential oil is an excellent one since it is non-toxic, non-irritant, and has been used to treat insomnia.

ROSEY TOSEY FOOT BATH

2 drops rose absolute or
    rose otto
2 drops rose geranium
2 drops rosewood
2 drops bergamot

Add oils to 2 gallons (8 litres) warm water and mix well.

This is a sweet, uplifting, balancing blend. Rose absolute or otto are a luxury well worth their price. Their antidepressant qualities can turn around a gray day, wrapping you in sweet-scented steam. Rosewood and bergamot are refreshing, analgesic, deodorant, and antiseptic.

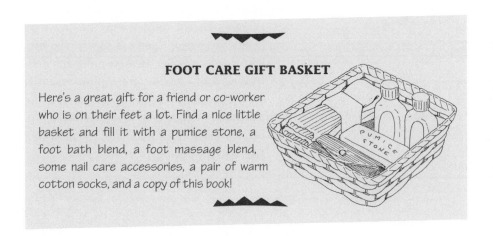

FOOT CARE GIFT BASKET

Here's a great gift for a friend or co-worker who is on their feet a lot. Find a nice little basket and fill it with a pumice stone, a foot bath blend, a foot massage blend, some nail care accessories, a pair of warm cotton socks, and a copy of this book!

AROMATIC FOOT POWDER

½ cup (125 ml) arrowroot (or cornstarch, clay, baking soda, or an equal part blend of these)
8 drops essential oils of your choice (see suggestions below)

To make: Combine the arrowroot and essential oil, crushing the small clumps of oil between your fingers to evenly distribute them. This is made only with pure essential oils; no base oil is added. Be sure to wash your hands after handling pure essential oils to avoid any contact with the eyes or delicate mucous membranes.

Suggested oils: Any of the foot bath recipe blends, or cypress, pine, juniper, ylang-ylang, grapefruit, rosewood, and frankincense are all suitable.

To store: Find an airtight container, preferable with a closeable shaker top. An old baby powder bottle works well; old shaker-top spice jars or tins also will work. Pry off the top, add the powder, then replace the top.

To use: Aromatic foot powder is nice sprinkled in socks, tennis shoes, and boots to keep feet dry and cozy. It also complements the healing power of aromatic foot baths and massage oils. Powder is good to use after a foot soak when not using a massage oil afterwards. The massage oils tend to moisten the feet while the powders keeps them dry. Needless to say, the aromatic foot powder is also great for controlling foot odor. Cypress pure essential oil is especially useful for sweaty feet. Its astringent, deodorant, antispasmodic properties make it an excellent addition to a foot bath or powder.

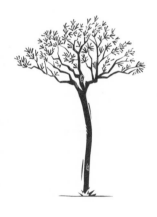

HAND AND NAIL CARE

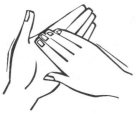 Being an avid herb gardener and crafter, my hands stay busy all day long. They often are roughed up a bit by digging in the earth, which also dries them out. Cutting and bunching fresh herbs and stripping dried leaves from the stalks take their toll as well. Whenever possible, I love to mix my blends with my hands. This leads to a lot of hand-washing, which further dries the skin and nails. I rarely wear gloves because I like to "feel" my work. (However, I do wear them when doing very rough work such as moving bricks around the paths in the herb garden, bunching up last years garden debris, or pruning my precious rose bushes.)

Despite all this abuse, people often look at my hands and say, "Those aren't the hands and nails of a gardener." Just because you work your hands hard, they shouldn't have to show it. I'm reminded of the scene in "Gone With The Wind" when Scarlett O'Hara's struggle to save her beloved Tara is betrayed to Rhett Butler when he sees the condition of her hands and says, "Those are not the hands of a lady!"

Protecting Your Hands

The first line of defense against worn-looking hands is a good-quality liquid castile soap and a natural bristle nail brush. I keep a bottle of aromatic hand soap at every sink of my home, with a good-quality nail brush in a dish nearby. I also keep a bottle on the utility sink in the basement so that I can cleanse my hands immediately after performing such tasks as changing cat litter boxes or scrubbing out old plant pots.

Adding essential oils to the soap helps disinfect hands and strengthen nails. Regularly brushing the hands stimulates circulation and removes debris under the nails where it can become lodged and lead to nail bed infections.

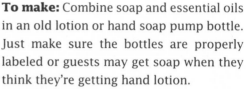

AROMATIC HAND SOAP

One 4-ounce bottle of high-quality liquid castile soap (such as Dr. Bronner's super mild baby castile)

40 drops of up to four essential oils of your choice

To make: Combine soap and essential oils in an old lotion or hand soap pump bottle. Just make sure the bottles are properly labeled or guests may get soap when they think they're getting hand lotion.

Suggested oils: The pure essential oils I prefer are lemon, lavender, juniper, rosemary, eucalyptus, pine, bergamot, sweet orange and grapefruit, tea tree, and clary sage.

To use: Add a pump or two of soap to a moistened nail brush and work up a nice lather, then rinse thoroughly. Push the cuticle back gently with a hand towel. This is a high concentration of oils, but it is necessary to disinfect and much of it is actually washed down the drain with the dirt and grime. I find that the steam rising from washing with this soap is sweet-smelling and enjoyable.

Keeping Nails in Shape

To keep fingernails in shape I have created a nail massage oil. I like to keep a dram-size (4 ml) dark glass bottle of this oil with an eyedropper top in a pocket of my purse. Then I have it handy to massage a drop into each nail when I am waiting for someone, or just have a few minutes to spare — at least twice a day. The pure essential oils benefit the nails in a number of ways. (This blend is pre-diluted so it doesn't tend to destroy the rubber bulb at the top of the eyedropper as quickly as undiluted pure essential oils can.) If you don't have a dropper, just dab a bit on each nail. Another easy way to strengthen and whiten nails is to massage clean nails with a lemon wedge.

NAIL MASSAGE OIL

1 dram (4 ml) pure jojoba and sweet almond oil base
10 drops of essential oils (see suggestions below)
5 drops of vitamin E (or 1 capsule punctured and squeezed into the bottle)

To make: Combine all the ingredients and mix well. If you prefer lotion over an oily base, substitute your favorite unscented hand lotion or cream for the jojoba and sweet almond oils base. A lotion or cream with no mineral oil is best.

Suggested oils: My favorite combination of essential oils is 2 drops each of: lemon, sandalwood, lavender, tea tree, and benzoin absolute resin. The tea tree oil is anti-fungal and may be omitted if there is no nail fungus problem; then increase the benzoin absolute resin and lemon to 3 drops each.

Adding 1 drop of ylang-ylang sweetens the blend and aids in its relaxing effects. Adding 1 to 2 drops of frankincense, known for its cell-regenerating properties (cytophylactic), is an excellent addition to hands with ragged cuticles or dry cracked areas around the nail. Patchouli also enhances this blend if 1 to 2 drops are added for a total of 10 drops of pure essential oils to 1 dram (4 ml), or 3 teaspoons (15 ml) of base.

To use: Pamper your hands before bed by applying 2 drops of this oil per nail and 4 drops per hand, and massage in. The massage is as important as the blend. It stimulates circulation, and relaxes hands that have been busy all day. This blend works equally well on toenails.

For nail fungus: A nail fungus often appears as a greenish, gray area under a nail. The use of artificial nails can lead to this type of infection. Keep an eye on your natural nails (and have your manicurist do so as well) if you choose to use nail additions. Tea tree and lavender are two of the few essential oils that can be used "neat," meaning undiluted. Very few oils are used this way, but in the case of a stubborn nail bed fungus, tea tree and lavender may be applied, either together or individually, directly under each affected nail as follows: 1 drop, up to three times a day. I have seen this treatment clear up a persistent problem in just a week. Follow up the treatment with a foot powder or massage oil with similar oils to increase its effect.

CUTICLE SOAK

1 teaspoon (5 ml) liquid
castile soap
3 drops essential oil: 1 drop
each of lemon, lavender,
and sandalwood

To make: Add ingredients to a small basin or bowl full of warm water and mix well. Add 2 drops of tea tree oil if suffering from a nail fungus problem. **As an alternative:** Add 1 teaspoon Aromatic Hand Soap (see recipe on page 110) to a small bowl or basin of warm water.

To use: Soak in this mixture for five minutes to soften the cuticle and cleanse the nails. Gently push back cuticles with a hand towel or orange stick while they are pliable. This is a very simple natural alternative to the classic nail soak.

A NATURAL NAIL FILE

The herb known as horsetail or shave grass (Equisetum arvense) has a high silica content that has traditionally been recognized for its beneficial effects on nails, bones, and hair. The tall stalks that appear late in the year by wetland areas breaks apart in sections that are rough like a fine sandpaper or nail file. These are nature's natural files! They are easy to gather and store and make gentle files for broken nails.

Never gather herbs in the wild without first making proper identification. Without experience, plants look so similar that it is easy to misidentify. Never gather too near a road, as toxic fumes from passing cars may affect herbs grown nearby. Also never gather on private property without permission. When gathering fresh herbs, never take them all. I only harvest a third or less and always thank the plant for its healing place in my life and beauty routine.

HAIR OILS

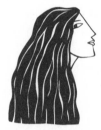

Oily hair! No, anything but that! When it comes to our hair, we've become an oil-phobic society. We wash, rinse, and astringe away every last drop of oil in our hair, then buy products designed to recondition it. Although I am no more a hairdresser than I am a manicurist, I do know what has worked for me and countless women (and surely some enlightened men) throughout the centuries.

Recently my teenage daughter, Christina, discovered the advantages of using sweet almond oil on both her body and hair. I felt a bit of satisfaction at this since the teen population is so particular about anything oily. After spending some of her precious allowance on hot oil treatments found in the local pharmacy, Christina wanted a less expensive and more effective product. She also recalled how much she enjoyed hair oil treatments on her long hair as a little girl that left her hair soft and detangled. Now we've revived our hair care oil treatments, at her request.

Aromatic hair oil treatments are fun to do, kind to your hair and help to produce a sense of well-being. They can be easily made up at home with just a few basics. I prefer a sweet almond oil and jojoba oil base. The amount needed depends on the length and thickness of your hair. The choice of pure essential oils depends upon your individual needs.

HAIR OIL TREATMENT FOR LIGHT OR DARK HAIR

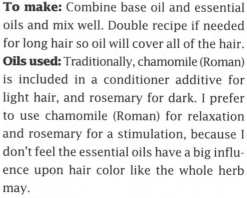

6 to 8 drops essential oils
½ ounce sweet almond or
  jojoba base oil (or ¼
  ounce of each)

To make: Combine base oil and essential oils and mix well. Double recipe if needed for long hair so oil will cover all of the hair.
Oils used: Traditionally, chamomile (Roman) is included in a conditioner additive for light hair, and rosemary for dark. I prefer to use chamomile (Roman) for relaxation and rosemary for a stimulation, because I don't feel the essential oils have a big influence upon hair color like the whole herb may.

To use: Apply oil gently throughout hair. Wear a shirt that you don't mind getting a little oily, or cover your shoulders until the oil is absorbed into the hair well.

Cover your head with a plastic cap or your pillow with a few bath towels if you plan to sleep with the hair oiled. Leave oil on hair for at least 1 hour.

To rinse, add shampoo directly to the oiled hair before you rinse or wet it. The shampoo emulsifies the oils, resulting in a much more thorough rinse.

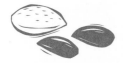

OIL TREATMENT FOR HEAD LICE

10 drops each of rosemary, lavender, rose geranium, and eucalyptus
2 ounces sweet almond oil as base

To make: Combine essential oils with base oil and mix well.

To use: Rub oil throughout hair. Leave treatment on for at least 1 hour. Apply shampoo and rinse hair well. Comb the hair with a nit comb after shampooing. Repeat the procedure in a few days.

Be very careful when applying oil near eyes. If essential oil gets in the eyes, wipe it out with plain sweet almond oil, not water. The water can disperse the oil too quickly.

If you ever have to deal with this common problem for the school-age population, you know how difficult and distasteful it can be to treat. Essential oils make a much nicer alternative to chemical pesticides.

SUGGESTED RECIPES FOR HAIR CARE BLENDS

The following recipes are based on ½ ounce of base oil. You may increase proportions as needed, i.e., double the amount of essential oils used for 1 ounce of base oil. To make an undiluted hair oil blend from any of these recipes, combine 10 drops of each oil in a 4 ml amber bottle.

Basic hair oil. This blend is soothing and refreshing to the scalp. Add 2 drops rosemary, 2 drops lavender, 2 drops clary sage, and 2 drops jasmine absolute to ½ ounce base oil.

Ylang-ylang blend. Add 2 drops lavender, 2 drops rose geranium, 2 drops ylang-ylang, and 2 drops patchouli to ½ ounce base oil.

Relaxing, conditioning blend. Add 2 drops Roman chamomile, 2 drops lavender, 2 drops sandalwood, and 1 drop jasmine absolute to ½ ounce base oil.

Earth Rose blend. Add 2 drops rose absolute, 2 drops patchouli, 2 drops sandalwood, and 2 drops lavender to ½ ounce base oil.

Scaly scalp and dandruff-prevention blend. Add 2 drops cedarwood (atlas), 2 drops lavender, 2 drops rosemary, and 2 drops tea tree to ½ ounce base oil.

HAIR CARE OILS

Equal amounts of the following essential oils: rosemary, lavender, cedarwood (atlas), clary sage, and jasmine absolute.

Variations: Other essential oils can be added or substituted, depending on your preferences and hair condition. Possible additions/substitutes include: patchouli, sandalwood, rose geranium, or ylang-ylang. The rosemary is sharp at first, then it diffuses and the deeper scents such as patchouli, sandalwood, and jasmine absolute linger.

This multipurpose blend of essential oils can be added to a variety of bases, including shampoo, conditioner, cider vinegar, sweet almond oil, and jojoba oil.

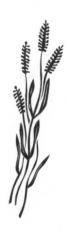

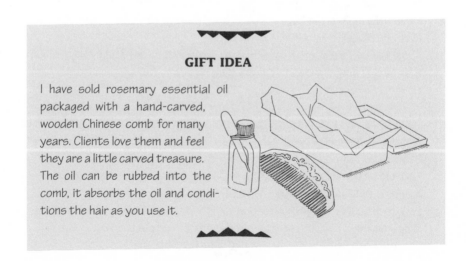

GIFT IDEA

I have sold rosemary essential oil packaged with a hand-carved, wooden Chinese comb for many years. Clients love them and feel they are a little carved treasure. The oil can be rubbed into the comb, it absorbs the oil and conditions the hair as you use it.

For scenting brush or comb: Add 2 to 3 drops of hair care oils directly to a hair brush or comb before using. If you have a wooden comb, the oil can be rubbed directly into the comb.

Hair absorbs scent quite readily, as you well know if you've smelled your hair after being in a room with cigarette smoke. I find I have to actually wash my hair before I can sleep after I have been socializing with smokers. I really resent it when someone lights up and directs their smoke toward my freshly washed and scented hair! One way of combatting these effects is to brush or apply hair oil blended without a base when in a smokey room. The oil also conditions hair as you brush or comb. This is a good treatment for both men and women. Do it for each other — the practice of brushing a loved one's hair certainly needs reviving!

I have a little bottle for my purse that I call Hair Care, containing a blend of rosemary, lavender, clary sage, patchouli, sandalwood, and jasmine absolute oils — pure precious essential oils can add a richness to any beauty routine. They are versatile, invigorating, and pleasing to body, mind, and spirit. This undiluted blend can also be added to a base oil or shampoo, conditioner, vinegar, or final rinse water.

To massage scalp: Place 3 to 5 drops of oils on your fingertips and lightly massage into scalp. In summer, try this while your hair is damp; sit in sun and enjoy being surrounded by aromatic oils as your hair dries. In winter, you can get some of the same effect with a blast or two from the blow dryer.

To add to shampoo, conditioner, vinegar, or base oil: Add 6 to 8 drops of essential oils blend to 1 tablespoon (15 ml) of selected base.

VINEGAR/CONDITIONER RINSE

1 tablespoon (15 ml) of your favorite conditioner (unscented, and with the least additives possible. Check your local health food store.)

1 teaspoon (5 ml) cider vinegar

5 drops Hair Care Oils (page 116)

2 cups (500 ml) warm water

To make: Add hair care oils to the cider vinegar or the conditioner, combine with other ingredients, and shake well. This mixture can be prepared and stored in advance without the water; add the water just before applying to the hair. You may also choose to use either the conditioner or the cider vinegar alone, but the vinegar alone tends to dry hair, while conditioner alone tends to make hair heavier and oily faster.

To use: Pour over the hair after shampooing. Gently massage in. Rinse, and towel dry. The vinegar scent dissipates as the hair dries and leaves the hair with a glossy shine. Resist the urge to use more vinegar. It is very potent and only a small amount is needed. I once used too much and after a light rain my hair smelled more like salad dressing than hair dressing.

SHAMPOOS

I've found recipes for many herbal shampoos in other books. They are fun to make, occasionally, but I can't seem to find enough time to develop a process that produces a consistent product. I prefer to buy a good-quality unscented shampoo and add pure essential oils to fit the condition of my hair.

HAIR RINSES

One of the best parts about washing hair is being able to apply a wonderful herbal and essential oil-laced hair rinse afterwards. The redolent steam churns up from the shower, enveloping you in a natural fragrant mist. The whole house smells good after one of these aromatic adventures.

I usually prepare my hair rinses as I use them so I rarely store them. My friend Elaine bottles her hair brew in old beer bottles. I have one of her tightly corked bottles with a wax seal in my bathroom. Trading creative packaging ideas with friends is great fun. It's always amazing to see what new twists different people come up with for making and packaging their own herbal products. Be sure to share your herbal endeavors with friends and family.

HERBAL HAIR RINSES

These rinses are made from the herbs themselves, *not* the essential oils. Essential oils may be added to these blends by the drop, but the proportions here refer to dried herbs in the cut and sifted form.

To make: Combine equal parts of the herbs in the selected combination (see following). Start with 1 tablespoon of each herb and see how you like the result. You can increase the amount later and store the blend, if desired. I usually store dried blends in dark glass jars. Fresh herbs may also be used, but you must increase the amount by three times to get the same potency as dried herbs. The essential oils are concentrated in the dried herbs and less is needed to achieve the same effect.

In a non-metal pan, bring 2 cups of water to a boil. Add 6–10 tablespoons of herb mixture. Turn off heat and cover pan tightly for 20 minutes. Strain herb mixture, cool, and use as a final rinse for the hair. This rinse can be rinsed out after five minutes or left on longer, if desired.

Herb combinations. *For light hair:* chamomile flowers, Calendula petals, nettle, *comfrey, and lemon peel or juice. *For dark hair:* rosemary, nettle, horsetail, red clover, and garden sage.

*Caution: If you are gathering fresh nettle, wear good gloves and be aware that it can cause a nasty rash. Jewel weed, which usually grows nearby, can counteract the effects of a nettle rash. I prefer to use dried nettle. It stimulates hair growth quite nicely.

Variations: Include peppermint, spearmint, rose petals, lemongrass, scented geraniums, basil, lavender, lemon verbena, or lemon balm. The hair rinse combinations can also be added in either fresh or dried form to 2 cups of cider vinegar. Use 2 teaspoons of the herbal vinegar added to 2 cups water for a final rinse.

PERSONAL PERFUMES

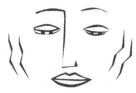 Perfume has intrigued man, and surely woman, for centuries. The word perfume is from the Latin *per* (through) and *fumum* (smoke or by fire), referring to the fact that perfumes were originally incense-type mixtures that were offered up to the gods to sweeten one's prayers. Deriving pleasure from scents is an ancient practice and crosses almost every culture. Originally, perfumes were concocted from natural ingredients.

Most modern perfumes, however, are made primarily of synthetic aromatic chemicals. These aromatic chemicals do not have the power to move us the way pure essential oil blends do. The components of anything applied to the body is absorbed by it. This in itself should make us cautious about what we use. I believe the advent of synthetic aromatic chemicals was in response to popular demand for consistency, price control, and supply. Manufacturers couldn't rely upon the graces of nature for producing mass quantities of their products inexpensively. The Chinese believed that every perfume is a medicine. I am sure this refers to natural perfumes, and hints at aromatherapy.

 A detailed and entertaining history of perfumes, including the bottles, can be found in a wonderful book entitled, *Fragrance, The Story of Perfume from Cleopatra to Chanel,* by Edwin T. Morris. The intriguing story this book weaves assures us that pure essential oils have played an important role in human life since the beginning of time, right up to today. People from every walk of life share one common thread: we like good smells and dislike bad ones. It's that simple.

I have been stopped in public on several occasions and asked by a passer-by, "What is that marvelous scent you are wearing?" This question often comes from a gentleman who is inquiring how to acquire this scent for his wife or loved one. At that point, I have to stop and take personal inventory to figure out what they are smelling. I may have been bottling pure essential oils that day, or working with some other herbal and aromatic substances that may have clung to my clothing. On other occasions the passer-by may be experiencing one of my homemade perfumes that I put together just for me.

Natural perfume-making is fun to do, and the rewards are wonderful, aromatic substances that enhance the quality of life, instead of synthetic aromatic chemicals that often fade out to somewhat less of a scent than one had hoped for. It can also be economical. Often most of the price you're paying for a commercial perfume is for the bottle, packaging, and promotion of the product.

Assessing Your Scent Likes and Dislikes

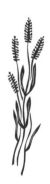

I recall having a keen interest in perfumes early in my life. My first true love once asked me which perfume I would like for Christmas. I gave him a long list, hoping to acquire a few to test on him. Much to my delight, he presented me with bottles of all those I had listed. I felt like a queen, having all of those luscious fragrances with which to surround myself. This experience instilled in me a love of aromatic substances that I know will last a lifetime.

Throughout the years, very few perfumes have held my interest. They always seemed to lack depth and staying power. I don't like smelling like everyone else, although the perfume ads promised you won't. Each person's own personal chemistry interacts with the scents we wear in various ways. I have often wondered just exactly why and how we choose a certain scent. I conduct a workshop called, "Own Your Own Aroma," in which we explore just that.

I ask the participants to consider these questions:

◆ How did you choose the perfume or fragrance you wear?
◆ Is it one you chose or did your husband, wife, or lover choose it for you?
◆ What exactly do you like about that scent? What would you change if you could?
◆ What are your scent preferences? Do herbal, woodsy, floral, citrus, earthy, or fruity scents appeal to you the most?
◆ Where do you apply your perfume? Does it last as long as you would like it to?
◆ Did you buy it for its fragrance or does that pretty bottle just look nice on your dressing table?
◆ Do you prefer different scents for the changing seasons? Do

your scent moods change with your emotional ones?
◆ Do you have a number of scents or are you loyal to a particular one?
◆ Would you like the idea of your personal perfume to help reduce stress or enhance your attractiveness?
◆ How would you like to be able to blend other personal care products to match your preferred scents?
◆ Do you prefer an alcohol or oil base?

These questions are a good starting point for natural, personal perfume making.

SUPPLIES FOR PERFUME-MAKING

For making natural perfumes, you will need a variety of pure essential oils, alcohols, and base oils, eyedroppers, bottles, a notepad and pencil, and labels.

Essential Oils

Perfume-making requires a variety of types, or "notes" of essential oils — including top, middle, and base notes. These terms used for the blending of perfumes correspond to the creation of music, since you're creating "a fragrance symphony," so to speak. The classification of these notes varies depending on who is listing them. The listing here is meant to be just a simple guide line. For a more detailed analysis, refer to Robert Tisserand's, *The Art of Aromatherapy,* (see Appendix), which has charts listing notes, odor intensity, evaporation rates, and a volatility index.

You do not need to stick to any hard, fast rules to create a perfume. However, a working knowledge of pure essential oils and their individual scents is helpful. I started blending perfumes by adding essential oils to already existing perfumes to enhance their fragrance. Although this was not a true natural perfume, it was a beginning.

Top notes. These are the scents you notice first. They are sharp, but they do not last very long. Moreover, these essential oils account for a small percentage of the final blend. Top notes include: bergamot, lemon, orange, peppermint, chamomile, lime, lemongrass.

Middle notes. These are added to smooth out a blend. These usually form the body of a blend and are used in a higher concentration. Middle notes include: rosewood, lavender, rose geranium, ylang-ylang.

Base notes. These oils add fullness to a blend — the scent that lasts longest. They are deep and earthy scents. These oils are often referred to as fixatives, as they tend to fix the scent and make it last longer on the skin although they account for a very small proportion of the blend. Base notes include: patchouli, sandalwood, vetiver, frankincense, myrrh, and labdanum.

In general, citrus oils lend a fruity note, spice oils a spicy one, and florals can sweeten a blend. The herbal oils add a green note and the root oils deepen a blend. For formula ideas on developing more sensuous blends, consult a fun little book that I picked up in England entitled, *Aromatics* by Valerie Ann Worwood (see Appendix). It includes drop-by-drop recipes and some interesting information that few other publications address.

The possibilities are limited only by your imagination and, of course, your budget!

Blending Perfumes

There are many good references on blending in some of the aromatherapy publications listed in the Appendix (see page 143). The scents one likes play a very important part in knowing where to start in blending a personal perfume. Experimentation is the best way to experience the marvelous scents that can be created. Blend one drop at a time. You can always add more, but you can't remove an oil, and may ruin a blend trying to cover up a mistake. Oils such as ylang-ylang are very odor intense and can quickly overpower a blend.

There are a few different methods for blending. Some people prefer to blend the pure essential oils together first, and then add them to the base. Others prefer to add essential oils to the base drop by drop, testing the blend as they go. Choose the method that works best for you.

Be sure to keep track of your recipes and be brave enough to try variations on them. How do you think Coco Chanel got to Chanel No. 5? I would guess that she had to go through numbers 1–4 first. Naming your perfume blends can be fun. Many a celebrity has lent their name to a fragrance, so why shouldn't you? Be creative and, most of all, have fun!

Selecting a Base

There are several bases you can use for perfume-making, depending on if you like a liquid or oil base. I prefer an oil base on my skin, but make an alcohol-base scent to spray on my clothes and in my hair. Natural perfumemakers debate what is the best alcohol base. I prefer to use Evercleer, a pure grain alcohol (95 percent alcohol, or 190 proof). It is unavailable in some states, however. Vodka is the next best thing.

I often make spice or vanilla alcohol to add to my perfumes. To do this, simply add a whole vanilla bean or 2 tablespoons of spices (allspice, cloves, cinnamon, star anise, and ginger) to a pint of Evercleer or Vodka. Let this mixture sit for 4 weeks. The resulting alcohol lends a warm spicy note to a perfume. It is similar to an herbal tincture in that the alcohol extracts the scent from the vanilla or spices just as it extracts the healing substances in herbs.

You could simply add the pure essential oils of spices directly to the alcohol. I find the scented alcohol more subtle in fragrance, and prefer it over the pure essential oils that can be so overpowering. If you choose to use the pure essential oils, please use caution as some of the spice oils such as clove and cinnamon can be irritating to sensitive skin.

If you choose an oil base, jojoba oil is a good choice. Jojoba is actually a liquid wax that doesn't go rancid as quickly as some of the other base oils. It is kind to the skin and hair. It applies nicely to the skin and tends to last longer.

Bottling

Pretty perfume bottles are enjoying a comeback and you will probably be able to find a nice selection. I have a little 1-ounce cut-glass bottle a young lady gave me one year for Christmas. It was very inexpensive and I have gotten a lot of use from it. Bottles with a bulb-type top are perfect for alcohol-base perfumes. For oil-base ones, stick to the dark glass bottles that you use for other blends such as massage oils and nail oils. A 4 ml dropper top bottle is perfect.

A personal perfume is a most welcome gift — one that says your perfumes should be as unique as your personality. I warn you, though, playing with perfume-making can become addictive and you will never look at (or smell) store-bought perfumes quite the same way ever again. I have made perfumes for teachers, stressed-out executives, busy homemakers, and lively teenagers.

RECIPES FOR PERSONAL PERFUME BLENDS

Here are formulas for some of my favorite blends. Remember, each individual has his or her own preferences, and experimentation is the key to finding the oils that suit you best.

I suggest adding the essential oils to the bottle first, then adding the alcohol. I have found that if I add more oils after I have added the alcohol, the blend may become cloudy. If this doesn't matter to you, blend away.

If you don't use the scented alcohol, then 1–2 drops of the preferred essential oil may be added. For example, when making the CKD I blend, I may add 1–2 drops of vanilla oleoresin instead of the scented alcohol.

No one has ever complained about an allergy to a natural perfume that I have produced, although I often hear people complain about allergic reactions to synthetic versions. I personally believe the allergic reaction may be caused by the synthetic aromatic chemicals used in the production of perfume, which are avoided with a natural product. Alcohol can be drying to the skin, so only a small amount should be sprayed at a time.

CKD I
I love to spritz this perfume in my hair.

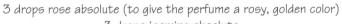

3 drops rose absolute (to give the perfume a rosy, golden color)
3 drops jasmine absolute
5 drops lavender
5 drops sandalwood
2 drops ylang-ylang
1 ounce vanilla alcohol or ½ ounce jojoba oil
(use oil blend directly on skin only)

EARTHY ROSE

3 drops rose absolute
6 drops bergamot
6 drops lavender
5 drops patchouli
1 ounce cinnamon alcohol or ½ ounce jojoba oil

GENTLEMAN'S DELIGHT

5 drops bergamot
5 drops sandalwood
2 drops patchouli
2 drops lime
1 ounce allspice or clove alcohol or ½ ounce jojoba oil

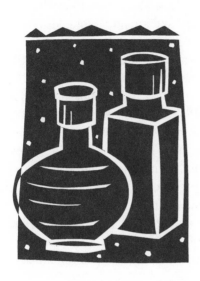

Other
Uses for
Essential Oils

CHAPTER

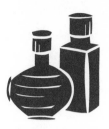

Pure essential oils can be of service in a variety of uncommon places. I have used them to enhance every place from airports to musty hotel rooms. Pure essentials have accompanied and assisted me on journeys into difficult situations like visiting hospitals and nursing homes and attending funerals. These oils have made the subways of Paris and London easier to bear on an unusually hot summer day and the streets of the city a little less scary to travel — my confidence and alertness enhanced by jasmine absolute and rosemary. As a personal perfume, essential oils have stimulated interesting conversations with complete strangers and carried thoughts and memories to friends and loved ones far away on aromatic breezes via the postal service.

Pure essential oils heighten my spirits and soothe my soul. They often announce the presence of a visitor before the person is actually seen, and provide fragrant reminders after they have gone. Through all of life's adventures, pure essential oils aid me in assimilating a variety of circumstances. They have the ability to increase beauty, reduce stress, and make a significant contribution to human experience.

MAKING TRAVEL MORE ENJOYABLE

Traveling can provide an opportunity to experience pure essential oils that you haven't tried before or to use old favorites in new ways. Long hot car rides can create cranky travelers. Carry a jug of water with a few drops of peppermint oil in it to apply to the face, neck, and arms with a washcloth to cool and soothe the weary ones. Lavender essential oil helps travelers to relax on long trips. In the car, carry a spritz bottle of water combined with a few drops of lavender. When traveling by plane, put a few drops on tissues and carry them in a small plastic bag.

Essential oils can enhance the car environment by adding a stimulating or relaxing influence, depending on individual needs. For a nervous driver, lavender may be of assistance. For a weary driver, rest is of the utmost importance, yet rosemary,

A WORD OF CAUTION ON TRAVELING

If you're traveling by airplane or into other countries and carrying essential oils, be prepared to explain what you have in those little bottles. I once had an airport security person mistake my wooden box of oils for shotgun shells on an x-ray and made me empty out my bags. I also found out the hard way not to stand around in a busy international airport inhaling deeply from little dark glass bottles. Security asked me to come with them and explain exactly what was in that bottle. I have never explained aromatherapy so eloquently or quickly in my life! This experience led me to develop a new product — travel tissues with essential oils that can be carried in a small plastic bag.

Custom officers are probably becoming better informed about essential oils, but don't count on it. Duty can also be confusing when importing large amounts of pure essential oils. I tried importing large amounts from England years ago and it was a nightmare. I'm sure it has become easier now, however, I only order small amounts from abroad and stick to domestic suppliers for bulk quantities. Larger companies have staff to deal with this much better than you or I can.

When you ship to or from overseas, make sure your pure essential oils are well packaged. I once received a lovely scented order from England in which all of the rose otto had spilled. I usually wrap each bottle in plastic to ensure that the labels on other bottles in the order won't be ruined by a spill or breakage. This is a great way to reuse and recycle plastic bubble wrap.

peppermint, and/or lemon can help brighten the senses. I put essential oils on a clay pot. After the oils have soaked in, I put it under the seat of my car.

I also create dash bags — combinations of herbs and oils that can be placed on the car dashboard and, with the heat turned on high, allowed to diffuse the scent. My friend Mary Lou used her Sniffy Bag™ (see recipe on page 25) when she had a cold but had to travel. Her truck became a sauna filled with redolent vapors that helped her breathe easier. After using it this way, she applied some sniffy bag refresher oil to revive the scent of her sniffy bag.

Air travel presents a number of challenges to the body. Take along a bottle of homemade rosewater to hydrate the skin and soothe the spirit. It also helps to drink plenty of water and eat lightly. Adding a squeeze of fresh lemon to your water can be refreshing. I have found that asking for a vegetarian meal on a flight, although I'm not a strict vegetarian, often gets me a meal that is a little more palatable. Drinking herb teas instead of soda or alcoholic drinks helps you stay balanced. I bring along my own tea bags and simply ask for hot water.

Jet lag can be eased somewhat by the use of pure essential oils. Acupuncture tacks put in the ears can also be helpful, by stimulating certain points in the body that are linked to alertness and balance. I did this once when I had only one week to be in England. Some people noticed what they may have thought of as my "new age" earrings and gave me puzzled looks, but the tacks did the job.

A massage before leaving and upon arriving at your destination can ease a long journey, especially when suffering from what I call "luggage shoulders." When a massage isn't available try a warm bath with lavender, geranium, chamomile, peppermint, or grapefruit oil. Grapefruit and peppermint are good pick-me-ups, while lavender, geranium, and chamomile are relaxing.

Pure essential oils are also useful in making yourself at home in an anonymous hotel room. One of the first things I do upon entering a hotel room is fill the sink with hot water and some of my favorite essential oils. I also wipe down the bed and spray some of my homemade perfume upon the pillows. These familiar scents immediately make me feel more at ease. Friends at herbal conferences are often able to "sniff out" my hotel room by following the vapors emitting from under the door of my room into the hallway.

CREATING A WELCOMING, CONDUCIVE WORK ENVIRONMENT

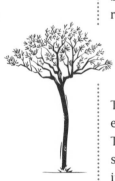

The way a place of business smells greatly affects the reactions employees, customers, and visitors have to the establishment. Think about it: When you enter a very nice-looking pub that smells of stale smoke and old beer, you don't feel much like staying to enjoy a meal. Grocery stores with the scent of rotting food aren't conducive to welcoming shoppers. I have been asked to do aromatherapy sessions in salons that reek of nail and hair chemicals, but I can't work in such a harshly scented environment.

When someone enters your place of business their first impression is made with their nose — a fact that most businesses don't realize. Think about the hours you've spent sitting in stale-smelling waiting rooms of doctors, lawyers, and city offices, and how they've made you feel. Then think about the enticing aromas of a coffee shop — even people who don't like the taste of coffee often say they love being around the smell of it. Or the toasty warm spicy scents that envelop you when you walk into a bakery, making you hungry for a goodie. It's no coincidence that the cinnamon roll shop at the mall is often close to the entrance — welcoming consumers. Even the astronauts on the space shuttle noted that the lemon-scented hand wipes they used enhanced the rather bland environment inside the shuttle. Movie theaters have known for years that blowing around that popcorn smell makes you want to indulge!

Use Inviting Scents

I know a chiropractor who scents his office with sweet orange oil. Sitting in his waiting room is much more pleasurable than the usual waiting rooms. Good magazines aren't enough to keep folks from becoming impatient. Olfactory stimulation can help people feel much differently about waiting for or even going to an appointment. Many people hate the smells associated with going to the dentist almost as much as the sound of the drill. What if the dentist used an aromatic diffuser to enhance the treatment room with the scents of lemon or lavender?

Perhaps a blend could be designed for the specific office, based on a scent survey of patients' preferences. The scent of almost any pure essential oil is preferable to the smell of bad or drilled teeth! The oils may also have the effect of helping the patient to relax during a procedure, especially if the patient were given the blend in advance with advice to smell it at relaxing times, thus developing an association between the scent and relaxation.

Selecting the scent for a business is largely a matter of personal choice. I've often heard it said that since all people don't like the same scent, it is better to use nothing. But you can do your own research to discover what your employees and clients like. You will always have a few folks who object to a certain scent no matter what you choose, but it will surely enhance a visit for the majority of clients and customers. I had a work-study student who was the nurse at my gynecologist's office. When I went in to the office under stressful conditions contemplating surgery (which I never end up having), she gave me a piece of gauze with chamomile, neroli (orange blossom), and lavender on it prior to seeing the doctor. This was an act of kindness that certainly made my visit easier to bear.

Real estate agents call me often to request scents to use in homes they are selling. Vanilla wins hands-down when it comes to scenting a home. People have actually called to tell me they bought the house because it smelled so good, and could I please make them up some more of the scent they love!

Introducing the Scent

Workplace scent can be diffused in a number of ways. Aromatic diffusers work wonders in changing a building's scent. These are now available with built-in timers that go on and off as needed. Carpet freshener made from borax and pure essential oils can be used by the cleaning staff. Tissues with a drop or two of pure essential oils or a blend can be given to individual patients or clients. One of my massage therapists uses a spray of pure essential oils to wipe down her massage table between clients.

We've just begun to explore the many ways essential oils could be used to enhance public environments. Schools all seem to have their own unique and memorable scents. Could school children learn or behave better in a room scented with essential oils? I have already had a number of teachers come to me for help in doing just this.

I have often wondered how essential oils might be used to alter the environment in prisons. Research has been done on the effects of various paint colors on aggressive behavior.

Could scent also be used to improve behavior in a contained environment? Perhaps it could help in facilities for the mentally ill, as well.

Japanese researchers are exploring the possibilities of increasing productivity and reducing error by pumping essential oil of lemon into an office building. While this raises important issues about manipulation in the workplace, it also acknowledges the potential effects essential oils may have.

Think about the offensive workplace smells that could be improved by the use of essential oils. The scent of a synthetically treated public restroom is nauseating and overpowering. The unpleasant odor often lingers in your nose long afterwards. The scent of an elevator crowded with people wearing synthetic perfumes and colognes can be an olfactory nightmare. Some offices and public meeting places are actually banning the use of perfumes. The subways I have ridden on in the world could surely use some aromatherapy! Buses and taxis could as well. Gyms and locker rooms definitely could use pure essential oils.

Take notice the next time you enter a building. How does it smell? Does this scent affect how you feel about that business? Then think about how your own place of business smells. Consider ways in which you might use essential oils to make it a more inviting, enjoyable place in which to work and spend time.

CARING FOR THE ELDERLY AND SICK

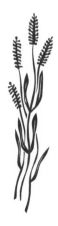

Pure essential oils can be valuable in improving the daily living of senior citizens. While the sense of smell does diminish somewhat in the elder years, the capacity to enjoy fresh scents (unless the sense of smell is entirely gone) never does. Bringing essential oils into the home are a way of stimulating memories and pleasant feelings for people who can't get out as much as they did when they were younger.

Ask an elder in your life what scents they have loved throughout their lives, and think of ways of incorporating these essential oils into their lives. I love speaking to senior citizen groups. They always have entertaining stories and aromatic memories to share that stay with me long after the visit is over.

One wonderful way for elders to enjoy essential oils is a refreshing basin bath. This is quick and easy to prepare. Just add 1 or 2 drops of lavender, rose geranium, bergamot, frankincense, rosewood, or sandalwood (or other oils of choice) to a basin of water and wash the skin with a washcloth. Follow up with a non-mineral oil moisture cream or a base oil with the same essential oils to condition the skin.

In the Hospital

Pure essential oils can truly help to ease the suffering, and improve the environment, for anyone enduring a hospital stay. The sense of smell can often be of service to our souls when other parts of our body, mind, and spirit have tired.

When my long-time friend Frank was dying due to complications of diabetes his loved ones filled his last days in the hospital and at home with hospice care with supportive people and pure essential oils. We massaged him with melissa, lavender, rose otto, patchouli, and grapefruit. He enjoyed sandalwood massaged into his feet, and dearly loved lavender rubbed into his beard. Being totally blind, Frank found the scents much more intense, and he was able to enjoy the fragrances fully. As I worked with him people would stop and poke their head in his room and ask, "What smells so good in here?" I call that the olfactory hook — it reaches out into the environment and invites one to enjoy the bounty of nature.

Before using oils in the hospital, be sure to check first with other patients in the room to make sure that the scents won't disturb them in any way. If others object, ask for your friend to be moved to a room where you can use them. In the hospital, I usually keep massage confined to hands and feet, depending on the patient's condition. When treating someone who is sick, it is particularly important to keep your blends on the light side. Remember: less is best.

It is my hope that one day pure essential oil will help in hospitals, nursing homes, hospices, funeral homes, and many more of those places that somehow linger in our minds and are often associated with negative emotions. Along with the antibacterial powers many essential oils have, they could perhaps make some of life's transitions a bit easier to bear.

In a Nursing Home

While acting as guardian to a wonderful woman named Mildred Bowren, I found out just how useful essential oils could be in easing pain and promoting comfort. "Ma" Bowren, as I always called her, had led a full life. She was foster parent to over 300 children in her career and ran a working farm at the same time. She and Frank Bowren were hard-working folks that probably never gave their sense of smell a lot of thought unless the lilacs were blooming or the smokehouse was full. Mildred came into my care after Frank died. I was one of the few young charges that ever sought her out in adulthood.

Mildred moved into a small apartment for a few years, but it eventually became necessary to admit her to a nursing home due to her health. Many people have negative reactions to the scent of nursing homes and hospitals. I decided to make Mildred's stay as pleasant as possible through the use of pure essential oils.

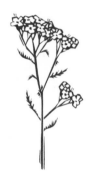

I started out by bringing home her laundry. Although the nursing home offers laundry service, her clothes could be line-dried and lightly scented with lavender for a calming influence as well as a familiar one. I had watched Mildred hang out laundry many times so I knew the scent of line-dried clothes was comforting to her. The association between freshly laundered clothes and lavenders dates back centuries when bed linens were hung upon lavender hedges to dry in the sun. When I hung her clothes in her closet they retained their fresh scent for days.

I also made lavender sachets to tuck in her dresser drawer (and asked a willing nurse to squeeze it every time she got something out of the drawer for Mildred), and stick it in the corner of her pillowcase at night. People have enjoyed the pleasant scent and relaxing effects of lavender sachets for centuries. This is another custom worthy of reviving.

Another custom I have always enjoyed, as did Mildred, is using rosemary in the hair — in herbal hair rinses, vinegars, and conditioning essential oil blends. Rosemary has enjoyed a rich history in helping keep the hair glossy and the mind bright.

Rosemary has traditionally signified remembrance. "There's rosemary that's for remembrance. Pray, you love, remember," wrote William Shakespeare. It was a treat for

MAKING A LAVENDER SACHET

Materials Needed:
A handful of lavender flowers
An 8" x 10" piece of cloth
(finely woven lace is nice, so you can see the
lavender but it doesn't fall out when squeezed)
A small rubber band
A 12" piece of ribbon

I call this my "no sew, basic, easy-on-the-herbalist" sachet. In other words, it's very easy to complete and a great task when you need to relax. Make several at a time so you will have them on hand as a welcome gift for a friend or loved one under stress. An occasional squeeze will freshen this sachet by releasing the essential oils contained in the little flower buds. These sachets last for years.

To make: Cut the cloth rectangle. Pile a handful of lavender into the center of the cloth (see Figure 1). Wrap up the sides and join tightly with the rubber band (see Figure 2). Tie a ribbon bow over the rubber band (see Figure 3).

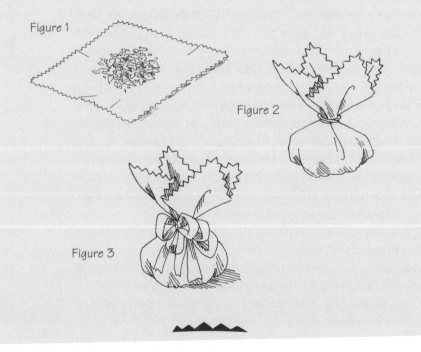

Figure 1

Figure 2

Figure 3

Mildred to have her hair done with a brush sprinkled with rosemary oil, and she always remembered it enough to ask for it again and again, although she was considered to be in the early stages of Alzheimer's disease. Research is underway in England on how rosemary essential oil can aid those with Alzheimer's retain and access their memories.

A pomander always hung in Mildred's closet to give off the spicy aroma of cinnamon and cloves. I wiped down her bed and bathroom with oils such as rosemary, lavender, rose geranium, and eucalyptus. I would add 20 drops of pure essential oils to a 16-ounce (500 ml) spray bottle and often sprayed the curtains, her mattress, and bathroom.

When I asked the nursing staff why pure essential oils — which are antiseptic, antiviral, and antibacterial — were not employed more by institutions, I was told that would be masking odors. When I tried to explain that herbs were burned in hospitals for centuries to clear the air, and how powerful an oil like thyme which contains thymol can be in keeping us safe from contagion, my words fell upon deaf ears, although their noses appreciated my efforts.

Additional things like peeling a fresh orange by her bed and sharing it with her gave her great pleasure, and massages on her arthritic hands and legs were met with deep sighs of satisfaction whenever she began to feel the effects of the lavender, rosemary, and juniper in almond oil that I used.

Mildred's whole sense of being would change after these times together. I know the quality of her stay was greatly enhanced by the use of pure essential oils in her room. I also think the nurses were so attentive, in part, because of how comfortable her room felt with its sweetly scented contents.

CARING FOR PETS

New information is emerging on pets and aromatherapy massage. One must heed even a bit more caution then when using pure essential oils on humans. For one thing, animal skin absorbs oils at a different rate than human skin. (For more on this, see *The Essential Oil Safety Data Manual* by Robert Tisserand, listed on page 146.)

Essential oils that have been found helpful in working with

animals to confront everything from flea control to depression include: Lavender, tea tree, chamomile, bergamot, cedarwood, juniper, rosemary, sandalwood, geranium, patchouli, sweet orange, and eucalyptus. The one essential oil you should *avoid* using on pets is pennyroyal. This popular flea repellant is much too concentrated in pure essential oil form.

Flea and Tick Control

Dried herbs and essential oils can be very effective in shielding your animal from fleas and ticks. See my recipe for pet powder on page 29. Keep pets out of the room while the powder is being applied and absorbed. I have seen a full-blown tick drop off of a dog onto the floor when a single drop of undiluted tea tree oil was applied directly. Cleaning pet bedding with pure essential oils helps repel vermin.

You can make an herbal bug-repellant pillow for a cat or dog by adding equal amounts of lavender flowers, cedarwood chips and pennyroyal herb *(not oil)* to the stuffing of a pillow or small homemade pet bed mattress. If you're substituting pure essential oils for the dried herbs, use only 5 drops total per pillow or mattress and, again, avoid pennyroyal oil. I know it is listed in many pet recipes, but I feel it is much too strong to be used directly on an animal. Also avoid using irritating citrus oils. While they are an ingredient in many flea repellants, they are used highly diluted. I once witnessed a small kitten go into convulsions after an unsuspecting owner applied orange oil to its fur. I would not suggest using pure essential oils with young puppies or kittens. I tend to use homeopathy with my cats and they very seldom have the need for pure essential oils.

Pure essential oils may, however, be added in small amounts to a pet's bathwater, approximately 8 drops of essential oil to two gallons of water. Eucalyptus, lavender, juniper, cedarwood, peppermint, or tea tree work well.

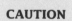

CAUTION

Always consult a qualified veterinarian before attempting to treat a pet's potentially serious condition on your own.

Other Pet Health Care Treatments

One solution I have found effective in helping to clear up minor cuts, scrapes, and other little irritations for both pets and humans is a tincture of myrrh. This is a highly astringent product, and it helped heal a very nasty abscess on my cat Buddy's side when he received a puncture wound from another cat. I diluted 1 dram (4 ml) of the myrrh tincture into 2 cups of warm water and applied compresses of this every hour until the wound was completely drained. I then applied tincture of myrrh undiluted to close and heal the wound and the place the doctor had lanced it to enable it to drain. I didn't apply the tincture undiluted at first, to enable the wound to drain before it closed up.

When Buddy had a problem with his skin, due to feline diabetes, I applied pure essential oils and herbal salves which were quite effective. I started by applying a 10 percent mixture of lavender, tea tree, geranium, and patchouli in sweet almond oil. I used this combination of oils first to eliminate any possible parasite problem and condition the skin. Buddy didn't take too well to the strong scent, and retaliated by taking a nap in his litter box. I then applied a 2 percent dilution of the same essential oil mixture in sweet almond oil for three days, twice a day.

Following the oil treatment, I began a massage routine on Buddy's scaly, cracked skin with undiluted sandalwood oil (3 to 5 drops massaged into his head three times a day). This was costly and truly worth it — and having Buddy smell of sandalwood was quite pleasant for him and for me! All of the bad skin

FORMULA FOR TINCTURE OF MYRRH

Combine 1 ounce myrrh gum with 4 ounces 90 or more proof alcohol (I prefer Evercleer or vodka) in an airtight glass jar. Let stand for two weeks before using.

This formula has been effective for treating both me and my cat, Buddy. Personally, I use myrrh tincture to clear up a cold sore almost instantly or to drain and heal an unsightly pimple as quick as possible. I carry a 4 ml bottle with me when I travel. I have also employed astringent, antiseptic myrrh to a badly bleeding cut, and witnessed its effectiveness at stopping the bleeding. And Buddy can surely vouch for myrrh tincture's effectiveness at treating his abcesses!

came off, leaving bald spots, and the skin began to heal quite nicely. I switched over to an herbal salve with comfrey in it for the last two weeks and Buddy's head healed beautifully.

Buddy also seemed to enjoy licking the salve off his paws. Remember that most animals will lick off whatever you apply if they can reach the spot. For this reason, you should use caution about what you apply because animals react differently to certain substances than humans do. When I used peroxide to clean out and aerate Buddy's abscess he didn't appreciate the fuzzy feel of it on his tongue one bit. In contrast, the herbal salves he licked off were made from fresh herbs, a much less concentrated form of plant material than pure essential oils.

Buddy has returned to his old self. He hisses at Rosemary, our other kitty, just as he had done before he got sick, and showed a return of his routine spirit. I can judge his state of health by whether or not he comes to bed. When he became sick he wouldn't leave the food or water dish. Now he has returned to keep me warm at night. He is playful, active, loves his catnip bag again, is gaining weight, cleaning himself very nicely, and is very affectionate.

For Further Research

There is much more to explore and discover about how herbs and pure essential oils might be useful to our pets. If you're interested in finding out more, a great book that has helped me through many pet problems is *The New Natural Cat: A Complete Guide for Finicky Owners* by Anitra Frazier. This book includes a source list of companies that offer excellent pet care products. Another useful book is *Cats: Homoeopathic Remedies* by George MacLeod, MRCVS, DVSM. He is also the author of books on caring for horses, cattle, and dogs as well as *A Veterinary Materia Medica*, which is a guide to using homeopathic remedies.

Bach Flower remedies are similar to homoeopathic remedies and can help animals and humans through the emotional process of recovering from an injury or illness (the internationally recognized Rescue Remedy). *The Handbook of The Bach Flower Remedies* by Dr. Philip M. Chancellor is a good starting guide to Bach flower remedies.

If you are a horse owner, you may be particularly interested in reading Linda Wilson's article on Carol Stratton and her Thoroughbred Therapy that appeared in *The International Journal of Aromatherapy* in 1988–1989 (see Appendix). This article by a leading crusader for horse welfare and rehabilitation covers the use of essential oils on horses. Carol has had amazing results in treating with everything from asthma to emotional problems at her horse rehabilitation center in England. Animals have a keen sense of smell. It only makes sense that they would respond to nature's pharmacy.

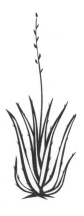

SOURCES AND RESOURCES

100PureEssentialOils.com
www.100pureessentialoils.com

Adriaflor
650-726-5020
www.adriaflor.com

Amrita Aromatherapy, Inc.
800-410-9651
http://amrita.net

Aromaland, Inc.
800-933-5267
www.aromaland.com

Eclipse Living Essence Aromatherapy Centre
enquiries@aromatherapyaustralia.com.au
www.aromatherapyaustralia.com.au

The Essential Oil Company
800-729-5912
www.essentialoil.com

From Nature With Love
800-520-2060
www.fromnaturewithlove.com

Frontier Natural Products Co-Op
800-669-3275
www.frontiercoop.com

Colleen K. Dodt
Herbal Endeavours
248-882-0023
colleenkaye115@yahoo.com

International Federation of Aromatherapists
+44-0208-567-2243
www.ifaroma.org

**International Federation of Professional
Aromatherapists**
+44-0145-563-7987
www.ifparoma.org

Kal Kotecha
Academy of Aromatherapy, Massage & Holistic Studies
519-885-6457
www.aromatherapy.ca

Liberty Natural Products, Inc.
800-289-8427
www.libertynatural.com

Mountain Rose Herbs
800-879-3337
www.mountainroseherbs.com

National Association for Holistic Aromatherapy
828-898-6161
www.naha.org

Original Swiss Aromatics
415-479-9120
www.originalswissaromatics.com

Oshadhi USA
Lotus Light Enterprises, Inc.
888-674-2344
www.oshadhiusa.com

Penn Herb Company Ltd.
800-523-9971
www.pennherb.com

Samara Botane
800-782-4532
www.wingedseed.com

Shirley Price Aromatherapy Ltd.
+44-0145-561-5466
www.shirleyprice.co.uk

Sunburst Bottle LLC
916-929-4500
www.sunburstbottle.com

Tisserand Aromatherapy
+44-0127-332-5666
www.tisserand.com

Victoria's Essentials
+61-3-9546-2225
www.victoriasessentials.com

SUGGESTED READING

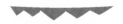

This list includes sources for this book, as well as selections from my personal library of Herbal Beauty books.

Ackerman, Diane. *A Natural History Of The Senses.* New York: Vintage Books, 1990.

Avery, Alexandra. *Aromatherapy And You.* Birkenfeld, OR: Blue Heron Hill Press, 1992.

Chancellor, Philip M. *Bach Flower Remedies.* London, England: Kears Publishing, 1971.

Cunningham, Scott. *Magical Aromatherapy.* St. Paul, MN: Llewellyn Publications, Inc, 1989.

Davis, Patricia. *Aromatherapy: An A-Z.* England: The C.W. Daniel Co. Ltd., 1988.

Davis, Patricia. *Subtle Aromatherapy.* England: The C.W. Daniel Co. Ltd., 1991.

Earle, Liz. *Natural Beauty.* London, England: Vermillion Press, 1993.

Fawcett, Margaret. *Aromatherapy For Pregnancy and Childbirth.* England: Element Books Ltd., 1993.

Fischer-Rizzi, Susanne. *Complete Aromatherapy Handbook.* New York, NY: Sterling Publishing Co. Inc., 1990.

Frazier, Anitra. *The New Natural Cat.* New York, NY: Plume Publishing, 1990.

Gattefosse, Rene-Maurice. *Gattefosse's Aromatherapy.* France: C.W. Daniel Co. Ltd., 1937.

Gumbel, Dietrich. *Principals of Holistic Skin Therapy With Herbal Essences.* Germany: Haug Publishers, 1986.

Hoffman, David. *An Elder's Herbal.* Los Angeles, CA: Healing Arts Press, 1993.

Keller, Erich. *Aromatherapy Handbook for Beauty, Hair, & Skin Care.* Los Angeles, CA: Healing Arts Press, 1991.

Keller, Erich. *The Complete Home Guide to Aromatherapy.* Germany: H.J. Kramer Inc., 1989.

Lavabre, Marcel. *Aromatherapy Workbook.* Los Angeles, CA: Healing Arts Press, 1990.

Lawless, Julia. *The Encyclopedia of Essential Oils.* England: Element Books Ltd., 1992.

Maury, Marguerite. *Marguerite Maury's Guide to Aromatherapy.* England: C.W. Daniel Co. Ltd., 1989.

Maxwell-Hudson, Clare. *Aromatherapy Massage*. London, England: Dorling Kindersley, 1994.

Macleod, George. *Cats: Homeopathic Remedies*. England: C.W. Daniel Co., Ltd., 1990.

Newdick, Jane. *At Home with Herbs*. North Adams, MA: Storey Publishing, 1995.

Price, Shirley. *Aromatherapy for Common Ailments*. London, England: Simon & Schuster Inc., 1991.

Price, Shirley. *Aromatherapy Workbook*. London, England: Thorsons Publishers, 1994.

Price, Shirley. *Practical Aromatherapy*. London, England: Thorsons Publishers Ltd., 1994.

Rose, Jeanne & Alexandra Avery. *The Cosmetic Aromatherapy Book*. Berkeley, CA: North Atlantic Books, 1991.

Ryman, Danielle. *The Aromatherapy Handbook*. London, England: Beckman, 1990.

Sellar, Wanda. *The Directory of Essential Oils*. London, England: C.W. Daniel Co. Ltd., 1992.

Tisserand, Maggie. *Aromatherapy for Women*. England: Thorsons Publishing Group, 1986.

Tisserand, Robert. *Aromatherapy to Heal and Tend the Body*. Lotus, CA: Lotus Press, 1988.

Tisserand, Robert. *The Essential Oil Safety Data Manual*. England: The Association of Tisserand Aromatherapists, 1985.

Tisserand, Robert. *The Art of Aromatherapy*. London, England: C.W. Daniel Co. Ltd., 1977.

Tourles, Stephanie. *The Herbal Body Book*. North Adams, MA: Storey Publishing, 1994.

Valnet, Jean, M.D. *Practice of Aromatherapy*. Rochester, VT: Inner Traditions, 1990.

Wiltwood, Christine. *Aromatherapy Stress Management*. England: Amberwood Publishing, 1993.

Worwood, Valerie Ann. *Aromantics*. New York, NY: Bantam Books, 1994.

Worwood, Valerie Ann. *The Complete Book of Essential Oils and Aromatherapy*. London, England: New World Library, 1991.

Worwood, Valerie Ann. *The Fragrant Mind*. London, England: Doubleday, 1995.

INDEX

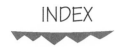

Page references in *italics* indicate illustrations.

Essential oils
    defined, 10
    elements in, 11
Essential Oil Safety Data Manual, The
    (Tisserand), 137
Eucalyptus *(Eucalyptus globulus),*
    24–25, 71, 73, 75
Exotic Evening Bath, 90
Extraction methods, 10–11

F
Facial oil recipes, 67, 88
Fawcett, Margaret, 16
Floor cleaning/washing, oils for, 71
Flower Toes Bath, 106
Foot baths
    caution when adding oils to, 103
    dish basin method, 101–2
    importance of, 100–101
    massage, 103, 104
    recipes, 103–7
    for sore or swollen feet, 102
    tub method, 102–3
Foot Powder, Aromatic, 108
Fragrance, The Story of Perfume
    from Cleopatra to Chanel
    (Morris), 120
Frankincense *(Boswellia carteri),* 47,
    84
Frazier, Anitra, 140

G
Gentleman's Delight perfume, 126
Gifts
    aromatic bath basket, 95
    bath oil, 89
    bath salts, 93
    foot care basket, 107
    packaging tips, 63
    sachets, 76, 95, 135, 136, *136*
Grapefruit *(Citrus paradisi),* 10, 26,
    73, 75, 84

Grapeseed, 18, 56, 61
Grief Bath, 91
Gumbel, Dietrich, 17

H
Hair care
    conditioners, 66, 118
    oil treatments, 113
    recipes, 85, 87, 114–19
    rinses, 66, 118–19
    shampoos, 66–67, 118
Handbook of the Bach Flower Reme-
    dies, The (Chancellor), 140
Hand care, 109
Hand Soap, Aromatic, 110
Headaches, 50, 51
Head lice, 115
Healing effects, 6
Heat sources, dangers of, 19
Herbal baths
    alternative methods for, 98
    bath bags, 96, *97*
    children's, 98–100
    recipes for, 95–100
Herbal hair rinses, 119
Herb Companion, The, 63
Herbs, use of, 79, 95–100
Holiday Potpourri, 74
Hormone replacement therapy, 37,
    38
Hospitals, oils for, 134
House cleaning water formula, 68
Hyssop *(Hyssopus officinalis),* 47–48

I
Inhalant recipes, 68, 86–87
Insect bites, 24, 31, 42
Insect repellant(s)
    oils for, 24, 33, 38, 46
    recipes for, 68, 138

J

Jasmine *(Jasminum officinale)*, 18, 26–28
Jet lag, 26, 130
Jojoba, 18, 56, 61–62
Juniper *(Juniperus communis)*, 28–29, 75, 84

L

Labdanum *(Cistus ladaniferus)*, 48
Lavabre, Marcel, 2
Lavender *(Lavandula officinalis)*, 10, 18
  description of, 29–31
  recipes for, 31
  sachets, 135, 136, *136*
  uses for, 71, 72, 73, 75, 76, 84
Learned-odor responses, 5–6
Learning about oils, guidelines for, 19–20
Lemon *(Citrus limonum)*, 10
  description of, 32–33
  recipes for, 70–71
  sun exposure and, 16, 17, 32
  uses for, 71, 73, 75, 84
Lemon Drop Bath, 99
Lemongrass, 17–18
Lightbulb rings, 59, *59*
Limbic system, 2
Linden blossom *(Tilia vulgaris)*, 48–49
Love Oil, 27

M

MacLeod, George, 140
Mandarin *(Citrus nobilis/ madurensis)*, 49
Massage
  See also Foot baths
  blending mixtures for, 90
  recipes, 68, 86, 87, 89, 90, 91, 111
Measurements, 64, 65–66
Medicinal claims, 17, 22

Melaleuca alternifolia. See Tea tree
Menopause, 24
Menta piperita. See Peppermint
Morris, Edwin T., 120
My Aching Feet Bath, 106

N

Nail care
  oils/ingredients for, 113
  recipes for, 111–12
  tips, 110, 112
Nail Care Oil, 45, 111
Nail files, 112
Nail fungus, 111
Natural History of The Senses, A (Ackerman), 4
Neurochemical experiences, 5–7
New Natural Cat: A Complete Guide for Finicky Owners, The (Frazier), 140
Nursing homes, oils in, 135, 137

O

Orange, sweet *(Citrus aurantium)*, 10
  description of, 33–34
  recipes for, 33
  sun exposure and, 16, 17, 33
  uses for, 71, 72, 73, 75, 84

P

Patchouli *(Pogostemon patchouli)*, 18
  description of, 34
  recipes for, 34
  uses for, 71, 74–75, 84
Pelargonium graveolens. See Rose geranium
Peppermint *(Menta piperita)*, 35–36
Perfumes
  accessing your scent likes and dislikes, 121–22
  background of, 120
  blending, 123–24
  bottling, 124–25